Trying to get Pregnant
(and Succeeding)

MARISA PEER

© Marisa Peer 2011 *26 January 2012*
All rights reserved.

ISBN: 1469942178
ISBN 13: 9781469942179

Front cover photo of Theo, Ella and Louis Pors-Campbell by Vijay Jethwa

© **Marisa Peer** January 2012

Advanced Book Reviews

Marisa Peer has helped so many women at Sands to have babies. These women found that they could not conceive again after experiencing the loss of their baby. Marisa's methods have proven to be incredibly helpful and very effective and I'm so glad that her book *Trying to Get Pregnant (and Succeeding)* contains her unique techniques so that even more women can benefit from them. Many Sands mums celebrate Marisa's work which has given them both hope and solutions when they have been going through their darkest days. For many years I have highly recommended her to Sands parents and I can wholeheartedly recommend this book to any women struggling with infertility. Marisa explains better than anyone how the mind can block conception after episodes of stress and trauma and her book shows you how to counteract this.

Collette Murphy, Sands (Stillbirth and Neonatal Death Charity).

Marisa Peer has been an inspiration to me in many areas of my life. When my partner and I decided we wanted to start a family, I was not just anxious, I was extremely unhopeful that it would happen. For many years medical experts told me it could be very difficult for me to get pregnant because of complications. I went to see Marisa and her inspiration, guidance and confidence helped me to gain the belief, assurance and determination I needed in order to get pregnant. I read *Trying to get Pregnant (and Succeeding)* and it gave me wisdom, insight and faith during many difficulties and obstacles. I am so glad I turned to Marisa as I now have a beautiful, amazing, adorable wonderful son. He is the light in my life. Thank you Marisa.

Daniella Neumann, TV producer.

I went to see Marisa before my first cycle of IVF after suffering several miscarriages and becoming quite anxious about becoming pregnant. Marisa was recommended to me by a friend who said Marisa had changed her life. I've never had hypnosis before so I had no idea what to expect. I was surprised to find how susceptible I was to Marisa's techniques. Marisa spent a lot of time understanding my background so that she could tailor the hypnosis to my specific needs, even using medical terminology in the session. I was also very impressed with Marisa's knowledge about fertility and all the latest research. During the session, I felt totally relaxed, like I was taken to another place completely. Afterwards, I felt ready to welcome our baby into our lives and I had a new confidence that it would happen. Our IVF cycle wasn't a success, but I fell pregnant straight afterwards naturally and we're expecting our baby boy in two months' time. I am certain that Marisa helped make this miracle happen. I can't recommend Marisa enough to anyone trying to conceive.

Alison Cooper, soon to be mum.

Marisa Peer has become internationally renowned for her profound insights when treating infertility using hypnotherapy. Her brilliance goes far beyond her early instinctive recognition. What has emerged is incredibly effective and she is one of a few hypnotherapists in history to have had a profound impact on the field. She has changed the field of hypnotherapy into something much greater than it had ever been particularly in the area of conception and birth. Her latest work *Trying to get Pregnant (and Succeeding)* is yet more evidence of her continuing evolution and profound knowledge in the people-helping professions. She has created a body of work that allows you to heal your old emotional wounds and this book is a must for anyone struggling with infertility or seeking to have a baby.

Gil Boyne, Director of the Hypnotism Training Institute.

I heard of Marisa when I read her 'You Can Be Thin' article in the press. Little did I know that this article would change my life forever! I brought Marisa's book and lost 14lbs immediately. The most amazing thing was that at the age of 38, I realised that I could 're programme' my brain to lose weight, I could also use Marisa's techniques to overcome my fears about having a baby. I brought Marisa's CD Easy Conception and was lucky enough to read *Trying to Get Pregnant (and Succeeding)* and within a few months I was pregnant. Now I'm listening to the Perfect Pregnancy stage of Marisa's programme and visualising my healthy baby growing. I continue to recommend Marisa's methods and 'magic' to anyone who has issues with becoming pregnant. Thank you Marisa for all the amazing things your books, CDs and powerful words have brought to my life. You are a true inspiration.

Lynn Harrop.

Before I read *Trying to get Pregnant (and Succeeding)* I was unconsciously doing everything I could not to get pregnant, by focusing on all the negatives (chiefly my age) and worrying about what could go wrong. Marisa's book has been an utter revelation to me, making me feel incredibly empowered. Before I was scared to hope to become a mum, yet after reading Marisa's book I think and act like a mother-to-be. I finally trust and believe I will have my own children – and it's all thanks to Marisa.

Samantha Brick, Journalist.

Praise for Marisa Peer's Fertility Programme

Hi Marisa,

It's so hard for me to write to you without gushing. I'll try not to. A great friend of mine has just been to see you on my recommendation and I know she told you about me and my baby Heather. She was born in 2001…I thought I'd send you a photo of her for your wall. She was born about nine and a half months after I saw you, not for infertility but because I had had a stillborn child and then a miscarriage (after two healthy babies) and had been told that I couldn't have any more live births. Anyway, you helped me feel so much happier and more positive about things and it really worked for me. So thank you a million times - and even that feels inadequate. (I told you I would gush). We went on to have another little girl after Heather, she is also very beautiful and I now have the four children I always wanted. I feel so lucky with them all. I always think of Heather as my little miracle baby and she certainly has a great spirit about her (that's a kind way of putting it!)

Congratulations on your great success on the television. It was a great and very pleasant surprise to see you on there. I wish you many more successes in your career. You really deserve them.

Best wishes and thanks again,

Mary Davies.

Dear Marisa,

Marina was born on 21st of April thanks to you helping me last July; I am convinced that your hypnotherapy session was the key to me becoming pregnant after a long period without success. My husband and I are extremely grateful. Please feel free to add Marina to your long list of fertility success stories. Thank you so very much again.

Lucille Shalaby.

Hello Marisa,

I came to see you back in April/May 2009 as I was having problems conceiving; I wasn't producing any eggs naturally and was undergoing IVF. Unfortunately, I never produced an egg in the three attempts at IVF I had around that time. But I continued to listen to your CD of our session and stayed convinced that I could conceive. The IVF doctors told me there was nothing else they could do and I should give up or use donor eggs. Yet within seven weeks of that diagnosis I was pregnant, naturally and without any sort of fertility drug. Bearing in mind it takes three months for a healthy egg to grow, ripen and release. That puts my meeting with you right at the beginning of that wonderful cycle that has led to the healthiest, happiest pregnancy I've ever heard of. I'm now nearly seven months pregnant with our son and can't wait until the birth (for which I'm intending to use hypno-birthing methods as they seem so akin to my 'new' way of thinking). I feel so very, very lucky to have conceived and rather stubbornly remain convinced I'll have another afterwards. Thank you for your help in making my brain shift gear, as tearful as some of it was, and for making me think of myself as a mother-to-be throughout the difficult times of IVF. I really am very grateful.

Susannah Dyer.

Dear Marisa,

I conceived all my four children through IVF. I consulted Marisa before my very first attempt and she helped me with hypnotherapy, visualisation, and mental conditioning exercises that proved invaluable. My fertility doctor urged me not to get my hopes up. That first time he was not sure it would work. He thought my embryos may not survive embryo transfer, but I concentrated on Marisa's exercises, remembered her words, and I became pregnant and gave birth to a healthy baby. On each subsequent attempt at IVF I consulted Marisa, listened to the CDs she had prepared for me and I became pregnant every single time straight away. I have no doubt that Marisa's input was a crucial part of my success in having and completing my family. Her caring but no nonsense approach is focused on achieving a pregnancy and having a healthy baby. I would recommend her to anyone contemplating or struggling with IVF. I am one of my IVF clinic's biggest success stories and I know it's because I used Marisa's techniques to make it work.

Helen Clapham.

Dear Marisa,

I love your fertility programme it's really terrific, so well written and so full of research.

I love "all healing is self-healing" – brilliant. Thanks to your pre-birth hypnosis I had the easiest birth known to mankind. I used your programme during the birth and had my daughter in just 25 minutes and with only four pushes!

Well done for a truly great book.

Claudia Rosencrantz, Television producer.

Dear Marisa,

I wanted to thank you for a wonderful experience with hypnotherapy. On Saturday I gave birth to a beautiful daughter Ruby, weighing seven pounds. The whole birth was a really positive experience. With no drugs needed, I delivered my daughter in less than an hour. You helped me enormously and I am so grateful. I am a convert to your methods now.

Much love and thanks.

Natasha.

Dear Marisa,

I came to see you for a session a year ago. I had terminated my pregnancy at twenty-one weeks because my baby had a serious heart defect. I was trying to get pregnant again but was riddled with guilt and fear that the same thing would happen again. After our session I felt at peace about the precious baby I lost. I listened to my CD every night, feeling more positive about getting pregnant again and it happened within two months. In March I gave birth to the loveliest little boy - happy, healthy and such a blessing. Thank you so much for your help. At forty-two I feel I have been very lucky. I had my gorgeous little boy exactly eleven months after our session.

Many Thanks,

Laura Davies.

Dear Marisa,

Well, you were absolutely right, he was a boy just like you predicted. My husband is even more impressed with you now. He was delivered a week early after a wonderful pregnancy and is the most peaceful, contented child, doted on by his sisters and his incredulous father. Thank you so much for our "healthy baby". We would not have him if it were not for you. I was told I was too old for another child and it was too risky after my last baby died. I could not get any help, but I flew from the Falklands to England to see you, and I am so glad that I did as we now have our wonderful son.

Our grateful thanks always,

Melanie and Peter Gilpin.

Dear Marisa,

A belated but heartfelt thank you; for all your help and support before and during my pregnancy with Victoria. You really helped make it all happen. I will never be able to truly thank you.

Louise.

TRYING TO GET PREGNANT (AND SUCCEEDING)

Ten Steps to Pregnancy and Motherhood

Unexplained infertility explained and overcome.

If you have eggs, sperm, a womb and a commitment to this programme you can make your baby.

This book is dedicated to my own wonderful Mother Dee Saddler who has always been there for me and is such a loving and caring mother and grandmother.

To my own miracle daughter Phaedra; who is everything to me and gave me all the joy of pregnancy, birth and motherhood that I cherish.

To my wonderful husband John for giving me endless love and support, you are the funniest, kindest, nicest most appreciated husband you give me so much love every day.

To all the gorgeous children in my life who give me unconditional love and fill me up with happiness and joy especially Carlyss, Lucas, Bree, Isaac, Freya, Lola and Jackson.

Special thanks to all my amazing friends Helen, Claudia, Dani, Charles, Jessica, Les and Glyn, and Maria and Gordon for reading my manuscripts motivating me and believing in me. I'm blessed to have friends like you. Thank you to all of my family, my amazing sister Sian, my lovely Dad Ron and Cissie. Heartfelt thanks to Dr Horsewood Lee for validating my methods and being so supportive of the work I do. Thank you to Sabrina my fantastic PA for all your hard work in helping me to put this book together. To the late Gil Boyne you are an inspiration and live on every day through your students who love you. You changed my life and taught me how to change the lives of others, I miss you and I am forever grateful to you. Finally a massive thank you must go to all of my patients for your stories and your generous permission to use them. You have taught me as much as I have ever taught you and I feel so privileged to share your joy when you create new life. This book would not exist without you.

Marisa Peer

Marisa Peer has had enormous success in helping women all over the world to conceive, even when they have been diagnosed with unexplained infertility. Her belief is that our subconscious thoughts and beliefs about pregnancy, birth, raising children, and how we were raised, can block our ability to conceive because of both conscious and unconscious fears. With a 20 to 25% per cent infertility rate in the Western world, which is not replicated in the East or in the animal kingdom, she believes that infertility is as much, if not more, mental than physical. Spending too long trying *not* to get pregnant can block the brain's ability to reproduce when you finally decide to get pregnant. One in four couples in the Western world will be infertile within ten years; yet one in three animals and couples in other parts of the world don't share this statistic.[1] Unexplained infertility is just that - unexplained. It is not medically based and can be overcome using the techniques in this book.

Marisa has flown all over the world to work with infertile women. She has helped women in their mid-forties to have healthy children and works with women to increase the success rate of in vitro fertilisation (IVF). Marisa also uses hypnosis to achieve a healthy, successful pregnancy, and a pain-free birth. She has appeared on GMTV as an expert hypnotherapist demonstrating the power of hypnosis for women during pregnancy and childbirth.

---

1 Lancet 2007, Guardian newspaper 24 08 2007

Marisa believes you don't get pregnant when you become relaxed about it; you get pregnant when you are expecting a baby. Not wishing or hoping, but expecting, knowing, believing, and seeing that baby on its way to you. This explains why couples in the process of adoption often conceive and why many conceive naturally after a successful IVF baby. They fully accept themselves as parents and see themselves as parents in every way. They buy things for the baby they *know* is on its way rather than the baby they hope or wish would be on its way. It's a little known fact that couples who are undergoing adoption are asked to use birth control, even if they have been diagnosed as infertile, because the statistics of adoptive parents becoming pregnant, even before the adoption has completed, are quite high.[2]

Most fertility books cover diet, vitamins, and women's cycles, and are quite technical. They focus on pregnancy much more than on actually having a baby and becoming a parent. This book is different. It's practical, and easy to follow and understand, and it deals with the role the mind plays in fertility along with a wealth of up-to-date diet, nutrition, and lifestyle advice. The cycle that makes pregnancy possible begins with hormones released in the brain and is directly influenced by a woman's thoughts and emotions. So as you read through this book, you will be able to change your thoughts and emotions, which can have a positive effect on your hormones. If you want to get pregnant, maintain that pregnancy, and have a baby, this book will absolutely help you to do that.

---

[2] Encyclopedia of adoption
Adoptive children and their families Proprius

Contents

Introduction:	Baby Blocks	1
Step One:	Baby Steps	31
Step Two:	Misconceptions	61
Step Three:	Baby Talk	79
Step Four:	Baby Rules	97
Step Five:	See My Baby	109
Step Six:	Baby Love	127
Step Seven:	Baby Goals and Affirmations	139
Step Eight:	Baby Food	149
Step Nine:	Baby Tunes	159
Step Ten:	Baby Shower	167

Foreward

I met Marisa after reading about her success with fertility in a magazine. My first baby Scarlet died and the aftermath of that experience was devastating for my husband and I. Life didn't seem worth living. Our only hope for the future was to try again. We never thought this would be a problem, as we had conceived easily when we decided to start a family. How wrong we were.

The stress from grieving had such a grip on me, both physically and mentally, that my body wasn't going to allow me that second chance. We tried unsuccessfully for more than a year following Scarlet's death. After cruelly losing our first child why would nature be so cruel as to deny us another opportunity? It felt like we'd never get there. A year doesn't sound long compared to some couples trying to conceive, but when you're grief is so strong, and your loss so heavy, it felt like ten years.

I was unable to see or even go near new born babies. I'd even cross the street to avoid buggies and happy new mums as the pain was too excruciating to bear. I then read about Marisa in a magazine. She is internationally considered to be the very best in her field and people travel from all over the world to seek her help. I generally thought I'd just give it a go. What did I have to lose?

When I met Marisa I was instantly drawn to her calm and composed demeanour, I'd never met anyone like her before. Her presence was magnetic and I found myself just soaking up her every word. I'd briefly explained my situation to her over the phone, so she was prepared for my initial out pouring of where I'd been and where I wanted to be.

I started the hypnotherapy session, it wasn't what I expected, and throughout that first hour I was fully aware of what was going on around me. Marisa's soothing voice and carefully chosen words instantly took root within my body and mind. I genuinely felt moved. It didn't really feel like an hour. I could have stayed for a lot longer. But that wasn't necessary. I entered Marisa's home thinking I may never become pregnant again. I walked out after one session, phoned my husband and said I'm going to have another baby. I even managed to speak with a mum and her newborn on my way home. Three weeks after that first session I was pregnant again. I felt like a different person. My whole outlook on life had been changed by listening to a woman I hardly knew, instilling all the positive words, thoughts and energy I needed to help me recover from the worst chapter in my life.

My husband and I now have two beautiful children: Freya aged ten and Dylan aged eight, and we couldn't have got there without Marisa's help.

Marisa has such a unique ability to help people with fertility problems to achieve the baby they long for. I have recommended her to a number of friends and acquaintances who could not conceive, and the results are nothing short of miraculous. For those people thinking this might just be a load of Hocus Pocus, they're wrong. Marisa really can help you get pregnant.

Now Marisa has finally decided to write this long, overdue book. I know there are a lot of self-help books out there, but there's only one Marisa. Getting pregnant is the most natural thing in the world, but if you're reading this forward, you'll already know that it's not always as easy as nature intended. Luckily this book is effortless to read, and Marisa's methods are easy to follow. It's like a session with Marisa, and you will change the way you think about getting pregnant.

Thank you Marisa for sharing your gift,

Love from Rachel and Mark Goozee.

Introduction

Dealing with Statistics

During the last decade, newspapers and magazines have featured regular articles about both women's and men's declining fertility, and numerous scare stories about how career women are attempting pregnancy when it is too late to conceive, reflecting a growing preoccupation with how many women are failing to have children. If you believe everything you read, you would think you have little choice but to have your children in your early twenties. In 2010, headlines in five leading newspapers including the Daily Mail focused on the 'infertility crisis', stating that the number of couples facing problems with conception is set to 'double within ten years', and that 'by 2015 one in three couples will need assistance to conceive, while many will be left childless'.

In fact, becoming pregnant and having a baby is something we can influence (up to a certain age) and is much more of a choice than we have been led to believe. Many women have had babies in their forties, including many of our parents and grandparents. Princess Alice, who lived to the age of one hundred and two, had two children in her forties, and that was over sixty years ago; yet fifty years ago, a forty-year-old was biologically much more like a sixty-year-old.[3] Not only are people living longer, but they tend to

---

[3] Biomarkers Willaim Evans and Brian Rosenburg Tufts University Ageless body Timless mind Dr Deepak Chopra Random House.

stay physically and emotionally younger. It is now possible to age in a way that slows down the ageing of your organs, so someone of forty today cannot be compared with someone of forty a hundred years ago. Their bodies and organs would have been entirely different and much older.

While nature would prefer us to have babies early, and while eggs can decline in quality and number in our mid-thirties, it doesn't mean you can't have a baby. You can use the power of your mind to influence the quality of your eggs and to understand the blocks that have prevented you from having a baby.

Most infertile women are diagnosed with 'unexplained infertility,' which literally means their reproductive system is fine, they ovulate, and they have good-quality eggs, so there is no medical reason for them not to conceive.

There are already many options available to improve your fertility, including vitamins, supplements, and diet. However, the most important tool for use in conceiving your baby is your *mind.* The human mind is the most powerful healing force there is. No drug in the world can match it; therefore any steps you take to conceive must be accompanied by a belief that it will work. Using vitamins, diet, and holistic therapies can only work, and indeed will work much better, if you also use the power of your mind and your belief system to convince yourself of their effectiveness.

This book will show you exactly how to do this. It is full of clearly defined, simple, workable approaches that get noticeable results. It will take you through a step-by-step programme that will change your beliefs and expectations about becoming pregnant, and as a result, you will be more likely to have a baby.

Controlling Your Thinking

Trying to get Pregnant (and Succeeding) will show you how to take control of your thinking, discover and

Introduction

change any limiting beliefs you may have about yourself and your fertility, as well as achieve your goal of having a baby.

This is not a book to read; it is a programme to use, so please do get a notebook (what I call a baby-book) to go with it, and write down notes and thoughts as they occur. Writing is very important - all successful people think on paper as well as in their minds. When you hold something in your mind, it is a wish, a daydream, a fantasy, but when you write it down and commit it to paper, it becomes more real, as you can look at it and revise it. Writing things down causes the conscious mind to accept them while the subconscious mind works to make them a reality, write out your thoughts as they come to you, and this will help you to identify any blocks about having your baby.

All the exercises in the book need to be done systematically and in sequence, so that you can receive new information and give your mind time to process it and absorb it before you introduce new information.

Working through this book in sequence will give you the time to change your thoughts and will excite your imagination and your subconscious mind. This in turn will make you ready for, and receptive to, changing-both physically and mentally. The ability to excite the subconscious mind is a great asset in boosting your fertility and changing your biochemistry. Scientists are just beginning to scratch the surface of the amazing capabilities of the mind and body, and one of their findings is that when the imagination is excited by positive thoughts and images, it sets off changes in the body.

Generally we absorb much more information in concentrated periods of forty-five minutes, than we do over several uninterrupted hours. Therefore, this programme has been designed to be read chapter by chapter, in forty-five-minute segments or less. You will learn and take in more if you spend an hour or so with the programme working on each step daily than if you were to read it all at once. If you can't resist reading it all at once, make sure that you go back and do the exercises day by day.

You need to commit yourself to doing the programme each day and to doing the exercises each day in the sequence that is written for you.

If you have:
- The *conviction* that you can have a baby,
- The *desire* to stick with and follow this programme,
- The *belief* and the *faith* that it works, and that you have the ability within you to improve your fertility (this programme will give you that belief),
- The ability to begin it, to *complete* it and to *follow through* every day,
- To *persist* in changing your thinking. Then you are much more likely to have a baby.

You may not possess these things as you begin reading this book, but you will certainly have them when you have finished.

Noticing Change

Since most change is retroactive and cumulative, you may not notice immediate changes taking place, but they are happening, so stick with the programme. We don't notice headaches going away, but we notice when they have gone. This is an example of change being retroactive. People notice they feel better, but don't notice the process of improvement. We see change mostly *after* we have changed, as we look back on our transformation, and it can be hard to pinpoint the moment or time

Introduction

when the change occurred. This programme is designed to improve the quality of your eggs and to help you to produce a perfect grade-A premium egg that will draw perfect sperm towards it. You won't notice that happening, but your faith that it *is* happening can improve your ability to conceive.

What this book can do for you is alter, in a positive way, the images and thoughts you have about pregnancy, birth, and motherhood, so that your mind has a different concept of what having a baby means to you. Many of these thoughts and beliefs are subconscious, but you can still change them. Changing our thinking causes changes both mentally and physically. We can actually change our biochemistry, once we know how. When you are making physical changes, such as when weight training for strength, the more effort you put in, the better and quicker the results. When you are making mental changes and altering your thinking, the opposite applies. You don't have to work or push yourself; in fact, you don't need to make a huge effort at all. Inducing mental changes is quite the opposite of the 'no pain, no gain' theory. As long as you are open to the possibility of changing your thinking, you will be successful. Thoughts can be adjusted in seconds-even thoughts we may have held for years. This book will show you how to do that.

This programme is simple, easy, and enjoyable. It just requires you to focus and to absorb some new ideas, to be open to change, and to be receptive to new possibilities. If humans were not already programmed to do this as second nature, we would still be living as primitive people. All the things I will be asking you to do in this book are fairly quick and don't involve much financial outlay. I will give you simple and easy assignments to do, but they are not, in any way, work.

C. S. Lewis said 'We are what we believe,' and it is so true. Our beliefs affect everything, including what we do, where we go, the kind of jobs and friends we have, and even what we eat and the kind of clothes we wear. Our bodies literally respond to our thoughts and beliefs, so if you think 'I'm too old to get pregnant,' your mind and body will accept this, literally. The hormones needed to make pregnancy possible are released in the brain and are influenced by the way we think and the way we feel, so negative emotions and beliefs can disrupt them.

The strongest force in every human being is that the body has to match what is going on in the mind. It literally has to act in a way that is consistent with our thinking; it has no choice. Every thought you think has a physical reaction in the body. For example, if you are scared, the body automatically increases the heart rate as it prepares for 'fight or flight.' Sweat and nausea might set it. When men think about sex they get a very physical reaction in the body because of that thought. When you think about eating, digestive juices begin to flow. These are all physical manifestations of what the mind is thinking. Thoughts are things, and they have consequences; good thoughts have good consequences in the body, and negative thoughts eventually have negative consequences.

Pain vs. Pleasure

Another very strong force in the human psyche is that nothing in our lives will influence us more than the things we link to pain and pleasure. Humans are ruled by these phenomena. When we experience pain the brain searches very hard for the cause of it and then it stores that information and does everything to ensure we don't go through that experience again. So some people can't go on a diet, even when they are obese, because they link pain to being deprived of certain foods. When we experience pleasure the brain searches for the cause of the pleasure and stores that information, too. For example, if you are shaken by a pregnancy scare and are then

Introduction

delighted to find you were not pregnant, this thought process can still influence you many years later.

The good news is, humans can choose what to link pain and pleasure to. Animals can't choose to link pain to giving birth or to being pregnant; humans are the only creatures who can do that. It is both a major advantage and an equal disadvantage. When you associate absolute pleasure with being pregnant and having a baby it's an advantage. If your mind links pain to the thought of giving birth or losing your figure after having a baby, it can work against you.

The mind holds on to outdated information if it has been repeated often enough. Every time you used birth control, you sent a powerful message to your mind: *I don't want to be pregnant. I don't want a baby*. Every time you took your pill, inserted the cap, or used a condom, your brain got the message loud and clear. If you have ever experienced a pregnancy scare you know that in that moment you linked absolute pain and fear to being pregnant.

I remember vividly praying for my period to arrive when I was eighteen, fearing I might be pregnant, believing I had ruined my life, and my parents would be furious. I was linking images of pain, shame, horror, and failure, to being pregnant. I remember being in our family bathroom sitting with my head pressed against the cool wall tiles wondering how I would ever tell my parents. I tried to cry silently, because they didn't even know I was in a sexual relationship with my boyfriend. I was due to go to university. They were so proud of me and I was about to destroy their dreams. Later, my period arrived, and I was as happy as if I had won the lottery and already got a first-class degree. The pleasure I linked to *not* being pregnant was strong and I was on a high for days. My boyfriend was pretty relieved as well. He was linking as much horror and pain to being a father at eighteen as I was to being an eighteen-year-old mother.

If you have been through this, you can see that you linked pain to pregnancy at an earlier time in your life. Of course years later, you want a baby, and now you are ready, but the mind does not always switch back after so many years of conditioning. Trying not to get pregnant for many years can be the greatest handicap to becoming pregnant. How many times do you think you have said to your partner 'Use a condom I don't want to get pregnant,' or 'Be careful; I don't want a baby?' Your mind took that literally, not just at that moment but for the future. The mind has a powerful control over the body, so every time you said things like 'I can't afford to have a baby now,' or 'It's not the right time in my career for children,' you told your mind you don't want a baby, and your body responded to that instruction. These words subconsciously told your body that a baby was not what you want and your body responded by not creating one. But your body does not know when you have changed your mind, and the old words are no longer applicable. This thought process is not automatically reversed. However, hypnosis is amazing at reversing it and much of the wording in this book, together with the repetition of some words and ideas are designed to reverse outdated thinking.

Very shortly after I had that fearful moment when I thought I was pregnant, I began having periods every two weeks. Then a year later, they completely stopped for eight years. I was very fit and healthy, but was diagnosed with fertility problems. Later I was put on thyroxin and was told my thyroid didn't work well and that I would need to take medication for the rest of my life. Some years later, during a routine check-up, I asked my doctor how I could get pregnant since I didn't have periods at all. He responded in a very offhanded way, saying, 'Well, you won't get pregnant on thyroxin, and if you come off it, you won't get pregnant either. There is nothing you

Introduction

can do about it. You must accept it.' I was shocked, as by then I was beginning to really want a baby. Luckily, I refused to believe him, and at some stage in the conversation I told him not to tell me anything else. I would not accept that I wouldn't have a baby. I decided not to hear what he had to say and not to let it in. I did believe it might take me some time, and that it might be difficult, but I always believed I would have a baby one day.

At the time my infertility was diagnosed, I was an exercise teacher working in LA. By the time I had had the conversation with my Doctor I had become a very successful therapist and frequently witnessed in my own patients the power of the mind to overcome a diagnosis. I thought it might take me a year to get pregnant; in fact, it took me two months. I was thrilled to be having a baby. The horror stories the medical profession told me about what would be in store for my baby and me had no impact. I was told my baby could also have a thyroid problem and, like me, would have to take medication for life. I was also told she would have a very small birth weight. In fact, she was born weighing seven and a half pounds, healthy and gorgeous. From that moment on, I decided not to take thyroxin again, even though my helpful pharmacist told me I might die without it. I came off it with the help of a wonderful doctor, and I have not taken it since. I am fit and healthy and my daughter is now grown up and is perfectly healthy.

One of the reasons undeveloped countries have much lower infertility rates than that of most of the developed world is that they link pregnancy with pleasure, honour, and a sense of fulfilling their purpose. Young women expect, and are expected, to have a baby soon into their fertility years, and they do. In tribal society, young women get married and are expected to reproduce within a year, and in many cultures birth control is only used after having given birth to many children. In some countries, it is a matter of pride for a man to father a baby and for a young girl to become pregnant in her teens. Undeveloped countries have much lower infertility rates.

When I was taking my daughter lambing in Northumberland, it struck me that one in four ewes are not infertile, nor is one in four cats, rabbits, mice, or any other animals. If you introduced a female cat or hamster to a male, it would reproduce over and over again. Animals cannot choose to link pain or pleasure to fertility, and they can't delay or put off making babies or link pain and shame to it.

I wrote my ten-step fertility programme because of my own experience of being told I would never have a baby and then having my wonderful daughter. I have worked with women of all ages from many different parts of the world with all kinds of reasons for not getting pregnant. Seeing their joy at reversing that made me write this book for all the women I can't see individually.

Psychobiology

Trying to get Pregnant (and Succeeding) is not psychobabble; it is 'Psychobiology.' Psychobiology is a term coined by Dr James Braid in the nineteenth century. He used the power of his patients' minds to help them heal themselves, and his success rate was very high. *Trying to get Pregnant (and Succeeding)* is a unique programme designed to activate that healing power within you to enable you to conceive, carry, and deliver your perfect, healthy baby.

I made a point of studying and researching cases of people who had succeeded against the odds, including people who had recovered from incurable diseases. Interestingly, there were no books with case histories of couples who had gone on to have babies against all the odds, even though I have met many such people and consider myself one of them. I knew that the same

Introduction

techniques that were used to recover from illness could be used to help people 'recover' from infertility. The more we hear about conception against the odds and miracle babies, the more we realise how possible this is for all women.

Carl Simonton, an oncologist, and his psychologist wife Stephanie Mathews, were teaching visualisation techniques to 'incurable cancer patients' who had been given less than one year to live. Of their first 159 patients, 19 per cent were completely cured, and the disease regressed in another 22 per cent. Those who eventually did succumb to the disease had, on average, doubled their predicted survival time. I also discovered that in tribal medicine, and in Western practice under the guidance of Hippocrates, the patients' minds were extremely important to their journey of healing.

Until the nineteenth century, medical writers never failed to mention the effects of grief, depression, or discouragement on the onset of a disease. Similarly, they noted the beneficial effects of faith, happiness, and confidence on the patient's recovery. Contentment was considered essential if you wanted to enjoy a healthy life. I was looking around the museum at Bart's Hospital, when I came across an entry in a surgeon's diary from many years ago that has stayed with me. It read:

'The feeling that cannot find its expression in tears may cause other organs to weep.'

It was written originally by Henry Maudsley a pioneering English Psychiatrist.

Modern science has been able to control and cure so many diseases by the use of drugs to such an extent that the potential power of the patient has been forgotten. Awareness of the mind's powers has been lost, as medicine throws out all evidence that is not easily quantified or scientific.

I decided this programme was necessary when I realised just how many couples are affected by being labelled infertile. The statistics are between 20 and 25 per cent, but they might be higher because so many couples keep their fertility problems a secret. The statistics are predicted to rise to 33 per cent within ten years. You need to realise that you are not alone. At least one in five couples will have difficulties in conceiving, and in ten years that is expected to be one in three.[4]

Clinically, the term 'infertile' is applied if a couple has difficulty getting pregnant after trying for one year. Approximately 40 per cent of such problems arise from the female, 40 per cent from the male, and 20 per cent are unexplained.[5] Words and negative labels have a destructive effect upon your central nervous system.

Close your eyes and feel the fear that runs through your body when you say the word *'infertile.'* Now see yourself smiling, and this time say the words *'super fertile,'* recognise how strong and good this makes you feel. Words and thoughts direct your body, and create your physical and mental wellbeing.

Trying to get Pregnant (and Succeeding) is designed to instruct you both consciously and subconsciously, on how to get pregnant fast. This book will teach you the miracle power of your subconscious mind, which governs your reproductive system.

I have worked with many IVF clinics, because of the power the mind can have on increasing the success of IVF pregnancies. These techniques can be used in association with assisted conception and can increase your chances of having a baby through IVF, intra-uterine insemination (IUI), or intracytoplasmic sperm injection (ICSI). The statistics for having a baby through IVF are about 25 per cent (depending on the age of the woman. The statistics vary greatly between a woman who is under 35 and one who is older). However, the statistics

---

[4] according to http://www.encyclopedia.com/topic/infertility.aspx
[5] http://news.bbc.co.uk/1/hi/health/4118976.stm

Introduction

for egg production, egg collection, and fertilisation are all different, and significantly higher than 25 per cent. To get to the embryo transfer stage, you have already succeeded 100 per cent at egg production, 100 per cent at egg collection, and 100 per cent at fertilisation. Many of the women I work with are successful at every stage, but are unsuccessful at implantation after the embryo transfer. Using the power of your mind to connect with your unborn baby and to instruct it to attach in the womb, stick and to develop to full term can dramatically increase your ability to have a full-term pregnancy and to grow a robust healthy baby. When women begin IVF, they often believe it will not work, at least subconsciously, because when women hear that the clinic's success rate is 25 per cent, many assume that they will be one of the 75 per cent who are not successful. Women are afraid to believe it will work. They are scared to get their hopes up for fear of disappointment. They do not realise, and no one tells them, that in thinking like this, they are contributing to failure instead of success. Some of my clients have even told me that whilst going through IVF, they have actually been told by their consultant that it is more likely to not work than to work in their case.

I am amazed at the amount of women I work with who say 'I won't let myself believe it's working because I couldn't take the pain if it failed.' I always tell them that they *must* believe it's working, no matter what. If it doesn't work, the pain is awful, but it isn't lessened by believing it wasn't going to work anyway. It might even be heightened, because you did not do every single thing you could to make it work. You didn't believe in it 100 per cent.

You already know from reading this book that your mind must move you away from the things you link pain to. Linking pain to the possibility that reproductive medicine might fail moves you away from a committed belief in it working.

Trying to get Pregnant (and Succeeding)

You Gotta Have Faith, Faith, Faith

I also work with women who get pregnant and won't buy a single item for the baby in case they lose it. They won't imagine the birth or taking the baby home in case they miscarry. What kind of message is that sending to the baby in the womb? In the womb there is no sense of gravity, no light only dark. The temperature is always the same, and there is no taste, no smell, no touch, and very limited vision. The only developed sense is hearing, and this sense is heightened because the baby is in water. Our babies hear our words and tune in to our thoughts all the time, so making our words and thoughts positive has a positive effect on the baby. Being calm, happy, and positive is picked up by the baby-and so is being anxious, fearful, and negative.

I ask my clients who are too scared to shop for the baby to go in and buy something, maybe just a pair of tiny socks, as a mark of their faith that their baby is on its way to them. I ask them to put the socks somewhere where they are visible, such as on their bedside table or tucked into a mirror so that they look at them every day and imagine the baby wearing them. One of my clients bought baby socks and used them as her phone cover so she was reminded every day of her conviction that she would have a baby. I ask them to mentally design and plan their baby's room with absolute faith and conviction that their baby's journey to be born is beginning and will be realised. Many of the women I work with have a belief that pregnancy and motherhood is not available to them except as a distant dream. They avoid the supermarket aisles full of nappies and baby food, as it is just too painful. They cross the road to avoid shops like Mothercare as they find it painful to see women with babies. They have a belief that says 'This is not available to me, and it is so unfair.' When they see mothers with three children, they think, 'I can't even have one.

Introduction

Why not? What is wrong with me? Why is nature saying no to me?' They feel excluded from pregnancy and exclude themselves from situations involving mothers and babies. Some can't even be around their friends' and relatives' children.

In order to become a mother, you must do the opposite. You need to walk down those baby aisles, go into baby shops, and look at baby catalogues planning which products you will buy. Say things aloud, like, 'My baby is going to have that type of organic baby food, this type of traditional cot or Moses basket, that gorgeous waffle blanket, those modern feeding bottles, that soft, cuddly teddy, this bugaboo pushchair or pram,' and so on. In your mind, or out loud, talk to your future baby about the items you are going to buy for it. Tell your baby about the fun you are going to have decorating its room, filling up the garden with a sandpit, paddling pool, and toys, and putting the baby bath and all the baby products in your bathroom.

The British Medical Journal published a study where women who had difficulty conceiving were taught to replace their negative thoughts about their chances of getting pregnant with a positive belief that they would get pregnant. Half of them became pregnant. This was in sharp contrast to a control group who were given standard advice. In that group only one out of five conceived. So the likelihood of pregnancy increased from 20 per cent to 50 per cent simply by replacing negative thoughts with positive thoughts. In another study, at Harvard Medical School, a group of women were taught to replace negative thoughts with positive ones. Of that group, 55 per cent went on to have a baby, compared to only 20 per cent of the control group. You can do that for yourself, and I am going to show you how.

When IVF embryos are re-implanted into a woman's womb, she is told she will not be pregnant until another two weeks have passed. This is because although conception and fertilisation have taken place, the embryos have not yet attached securely into the womb. They have not yet 'taken,' so she can't assume she is pregnant. The woman often tries to ignore what is happening to her, because that two-week period is very difficult. She fears that it won't work, and that is the image that fills her mind. In her imagination she sees it not working. She imagines that the embryo is very fragile and that it will simply fall through her. All of this happens automatically. By contrast, a woman who has trained her mind will talk to her baby. She will see herself getting a positive result, see the baby firmly, securely and safely attached to her womb and see herself carrying that baby to full term, and going on to give birth to a happy, healthy baby. She will give herself conscious suggestions using positive words and positive images.

Once your subconscious mind has accepted the suggestion and images, it cannot tell the difference between truth and fiction, and it will create the conditions of pregnancy. I believe that if you develop a strong connection with your baby, in your mind, and if you become emotionally deeply connected, it is easier for the baby to physically connect because it feels that connection, and so do you. You will find a script on developing this connection and encouraging your baby to go from an embryo to a foetus later in this book.

Your egg, your womb, the sperm, and embryo all know what to do. The egg knows when to leave the follicle, and as it travels down the fallopian tube, it gives off a very powerful chemical in the surrounding fluid to draw the right sperm to it. The sperm also know exactly what to do. They are programmed to travel towards the egg and to break through the shell so conception can take place. The fertilised egg then begins a five-day journey from the fallopian tube to the womb, and when it gets there, it knows how to attach itself and bury itself into the womb lining so that implantation takes place and the embryo is

Introduction

fastened securely into the womb lining, where it develops for nine months. The more you can see this, imagine it, and focus on it, the more likely it is to happen, as your thoughts and images are giving clear instructions from your mind to your body telling it what you expect and need it to do. We know that our thoughts have absolute consequences and real physical effects on our bodies.

The purpose of this book is to get you pregnant, keep you pregnant, make you a mother, and enable you to have a perfect pregnancy and a gorgeous healthy baby. In order for you to become pregnant, you have to understand how your mind works. Only by understanding your mind can you command your body to give you what you want. At the moment you are getting what you *don't* want.

Every thought you have is an instruction, a literal command to your body. Your body listens to and believes every word you say. In fact, it takes those words you so casually use, as direct instructions.

One of my clients told me that she had 'joked' about being too old to conceive. She had described her eggs as 'past their sell-by date,' but when she realised that her words had the power to create her physical reality, she stopped immediately.

Another of my patients had bought a two-seater sports car because she was sure in her mind she would never get pregnant and was trying to compensate, to console herself. As I talked to her about her beliefs, she said, 'You know, you are so right. When I was planning my wedding, I asked my sister to be my bridesmaid, and she said, 'Oh, I can't; I will be pregnant by then.' She had just got married and was certain she would be pregnant by the time my wedding took place the following year. Sure enough, she was. I, on the other hand, worry and fret that I won't get pregnant because I feel so different from my sisters. I have always been the odd one out, the black sheep, the 'career woman,' whereas my sisters

Trying to get Pregnant (and Succeeding)

are homemakers. They all have families, but I can't get pregnant.'

This client was a very successful court lawyer and had recently come across a British study that showed that both male and female trial lawyers have higher levels of testosterone than the general population. She believed her body would not let her get pregnant. I told her I knew lots of women trial lawyers who had given birth, and she must know more. These women just didn't know that they were 'supposed' to have difficulties. My client now has four perfect children.

I ask my IVF clients to 'love' the injections they are taking. I tell them that every time they open the fridge door and take out their medicine, they should talk to the baby, and say, 'I am one step closer to you, and loving the process.'

One of my clients said she felt fabulous when she was taking her drugs for ICSI. She told me that every injection was taking her closer to her baby. She was thirty-nine when she underwent this procedure, and the clinic commented that her eggs were typical of a nineteen-year-old. They had never seen someone produce so many high-quality eggs.

Happiness has a profound effect upon your body. Recent tests showed that when newly-in-love couples were given a small amount of poison, their bodies did not react to it at all. When a much smaller amount of the same poison was given to people who were sad, unhappy, and alone, they reacted immediately and became unwell.

When we are in love, we are constantly being told by our partner, 'You're amazing, you're so great, I love you, I adore you.' Hearing these words has an effect on our immune system, and it becomes stronger. Hearing negative words has the opposite effect, and our immune system becomes weaker. At the Rainbow Children's Hospital in Cleveland, a group of children were shown a puppet show. One puppet represented a germ and the other puppet was

Introduction

the immune system. The immune system puppet, which was made to look like a policeman, fought the germ and defeated it. The children were then asked to close their eyes and imagine the puppets in their bodies, with lots of immune system puppets killing all the germs. This lasted for only a few minutes, and then saliva samples were taken from the children. The results of the saliva samples showed that their immunoglobulin levels had increased significantly. (Immunoglobulin is a protein released by the body when it's under attack from infection.) The children's immune systems had responded as if they were fighting a real infection, as if a virus was actually present, and they were stronger as a result, even though the virus only existed in their imaginations.

Scientists have irrefutable evidence that we can all boost our immune systems just by thinking about them in a particular way. You can boost your fertility and improve your chances of conceiving, carrying, and delivering a healthy baby just by thinking of it in a certain way that is more positive. Doctors already know that babies in the womb respond to their mother's words and thoughts, and some Doctors believe the high miscarriage rate can be due to some babies feeling, or hearing, they are not wanted, and consequently miscarrying. This is hard to hear for parents' who have lost a much-wanted and cherished baby, and of course it does not apply to all miscarriages, but it has to be taken into consideration.

Words That Matter

Ancient tribes recognised that disease is not so much in the body as in the mind, which envelops the body. You do not live in your body; you live in your thoughts and feelings, which surround your body. When was the last time you spoke to your body with love or suggested that it was doing something right? The words we use have a profound effect upon our central nervous system. Another word for disappointed is 'failed.' We want to choose fertility, pregnancy, and motherhood, and we can do this only by proper instructions to our body. To give our body correct instructions, we have to believe it will work. We have to have faith, confidence, and unshakeable certainty that this is going to work. The opposite of this is a different kind of certainty, a certainty of fear and failure, a certainty that it won't work. The words 'hope,' 'wish,' 'dream,' and 'if only,' are very different from knowing with unwavering conviction that you will make it work.

Close your eyes for a moment and repeat to yourself out loud, over and over, 'I *hope* I have a baby, I *hope* I get pregnant' 'I *wish* I could have a baby.' Then open your eyes, and notice how you feel.

Close your eyes again and repeat to yourself out loud, over and over, 'I *know* I will have a baby, I *will* make it work my baby *is* on its way to me.' Then open your eyes and notice how you feel.

Saying 'I hope' is giving the power to someone else, some external force, hoping and longing that it will work but not really being at all sure or convinced. Saying 'I know it will work, I will make it work' is taking responsibility for making it work, which gives you a greater feeling of certainty that you can make it happen.

Making babies should be the most happy and wonderful time. However, it has often become an occasion fraught with stress, anxiety and disappointment to such an extent that couples trying for a baby no longer enjoy making love, and women go into IVF dreading and fearing the process. Even the words 'we are trying for a baby' are incorrect, as 'trying' implies possible failure we don't *try* to go to work and *try* to come home again, we do it. Stage hypnotists always instruct their volunteers to try when they say things like: 'Try to open your eyes and find they are glued shut; try to lift your arm and

Introduction

notice it is too heavy.' This is called a 'misdirect', giving the mind contradictory suggestions, implying we can try to do something, but we won't succeed.

Don't misdirect your own mind by using the word 'try' for anything that you really want to succeed at. You are not 'trying for' a baby; you are making a perfect baby because that is what you are designed to do, and it's what nature wants you to do. Women who use the internet to search for answers to infertility type in the phrase 'trying to get pregnant' more frequently than any other. I chose to call my programme *Trying to Get Pregnant (and Succeeding)* because I so want to help all the women that use that term. But even now at this stage in the book you must abandon the words trying for a baby and and replace them with I am making a baby or I am having a baby.

You may be wondering at this stage how women manage to have unwanted teenage pregnancies but the very point of teenage pregnancies is that teenagers are usually completely unstressed about pregnancy they are reckless, careless and oblivious to the extent that getting pregnant is not even on their radar.

You are nature's miracle. You have over fifteen billion brain cells that together are twinkling with more circuitry than a thousand cities. Your ears can hear sixteen hundred different frequencies ranging from twenty to twenty thousand cycles per second. Your eyes can detect a single photon of light, and the eight hundred thousand fibres in each of your optic nerves transmit more information from 132 million rods and cones to your brain than the world's largest optical computer system. More than three hundred million air sacs in your lungs provide oxygen to one hundred trillion cells throughout your body. Your twenty-six bones and 656 muscles form a more functionally diverse system of capabilities than any other known creature. These tremendous abilities to function and learn can be applied in many different ways. You cannot count all your capabilities; there are too many and they are all governed by your subconscious mind. Is it such a leap of faith to expect that your words and thoughts would influence this complex communication system within your body?

Imagine that you are standing in your kitchen holding a lemon that you have just taken from the fridge. It feels cold in your hand. Look at the outside of it, the yellow waxy skin that comes to a small green point at both ends. Squeeze it a little and feel its firmness and its weight. Now raise the lemon to your nose and smell it. Nothing smells quite like a lemon, does it? Now cut the lemon in half and smell it. The smell is stronger. Now bite deeply into the lemon, and let the juice swirl around in your mouth. Nothing tastes quite like a lemon, does it? At this point, if you have used your imagination well, your mouth will be watering.

Let us consider the implications of this. Mere words affected your salivary glands. The words did not reflect reality, but something you imagined. When you read those words about the lemon you were telling your brain you had a lemon. Although you did not mean it, your brain took it seriously and said to your salivary glands, 'She is biting a lemon. Hurry, wash it away.' Your glands obeyed.

If something as simple as imagining you were eating a lemon can cause your body to react physically, something as simple as imagining you are super fertile and able to have a baby can also cause your body to react, because we are put on this planet to reproduce, and your body is geared for reproduction.

Words do not just *reflect* reality they *create* reality, like the flow of saliva. The subconscious mind is no subtle interpreter of your intentions. It receives information and it stores it, believing without question everything you tell it, since its job is not to question but to act immediately on your instructions. Our subconscious is in charge of our

Introduction

bodies. Tell it something like, 'I am eating a lemon,' and it goes to work. The experiment we just did was neutral, meaning that physically no good or harm can come from it. But good as well as harm can come from many of the words we use.

If you are on an aeroplane waiting to fly to New York, you might be filling your mind with images of the shopping you are going to do, the shows you are going to see, the weather you are going to enjoy, and you will respond to those images. The person next to you might be filling her mind with images of terrorists. She might believe that some of the passengers look like terrorists, and as she focuses on the fact that the plane might crash, she will respond to those images. So two people on the same flight are responding differently because of the words and images they are creating.

The way we feel at any given time is due to only two things: the pictures we make in our head and the words we say to ourselves. The good news is that we can change those words and pictures at any time, and we can learn to make them more positive all the time.

The Power of Autosuggestion

Emile Coue was a French pharmacist who was in practice at the end of the nineteenth century and the beginning of the twentieth century. He noticed that when he was dispensing drugs, patients always did better when he gave them positive suggestions. Coue reasoned that each of us has two selves: a conscious, and an unconscious self. The conscious self, which you are aware of, has an unreliable memory, whereas the unconscious self has a marvellous memory. It registers, without our knowledge, the smallest events and the least important acts of our existence. Your subconscious is also credulous, and it accepts without reasoning what it is told, especially what *you* tell it, since it has no reason to doubt you.

Your unconscious is responsible for the functioning of all your organs. If your subconscious believes that your reproductive system is functioning successfully, then it will be a peak performer. However, if it has accepted a suggestion that it is not in your interest to have a baby, then regardless of whether you are ovulating, your tubes are clear, and your reproductive system is functioning normally, you might not have a baby.

Any negative suggestions, which you may not be consciously aware of, can form blocks in your mind to prevent conception. I call these Baby Blocks. This is when the subconscious mind believes that conception or motherhood would be a threat to a woman. They are caused by negative autosuggestion, and the only way round them is by conscious autosuggestion. If your mind believes for any reason whatsoever that you should not have a baby, it will become the most effective form of birth control. Our unconscious presides over all our actions, whatever they are. This is what we call imagination, and contrary to accepted opinion, imagination makes us act, even against our will. It is an absolute law of the mind that your imagination always beats your willpower. Imagination is far more powerful than knowledge, and emotion is more powerful than logic when dealing with our own minds and those of other people. Most women who are undergoing IVF are desperate to have a baby, but in their imagination they see the procedure failing.

If I asked you to stand on a window ledge only inches from the ground, you could stand on it effortlessly because you would imagine it to be easy, and that you cannot fall to the ground, because the ground is only a step away. However, if you imagine that window ledge is now high up on the outside of a skyscraper, you would be scared of standing on it in case you fell to the ground.

Introduction

You would become anxious and nervous and more likely to fall off. You could stand on that amount of space when it was near the ground because your imagination told you it was okay. Now your imagination is telling you that it is not okay, you could fall and die, and that same imagination will stop you from doing it. Even if you were offered a lot of money to stand on a window ledge fifty storeys high, you would be unable to do so, because in your imagination you see yourself falling, and in this scenario your will is powerless against your imagination. The fear is caused entirely by the picture that you made in your mind and the words that you are going to fall. This transforms itself instantly into fact, because your mind cannot tell the difference between fact and fiction, in spite of all the efforts of your will, the harder that you try not to fall, the more likely it is that you will fall. Your mind cannot hold two pictures at once, so in order for you to think of *not* falling, you have to see yourself falling.

When you are trying to have a baby, you don't want to get your hopes up. Your determination is willing you to get pregnant, but your fear is causing your imagination to see it failing. It is the absolute rule of the mind that your imagination will always win.

Train Your Imagination

The aim of this book is to train your imagination, so that you will win. Your imagination is like an untamed horse, it is immensely powerful, and you have to go where it wants you to go. The problem is that your subconscious mind has been formed by suggestions given to you by other people, by the media, by things you have seen on television, read in magazines, or heard other people saying. You accepted the suggestions at a time in your life when you did not want a baby. Now, by learning and understanding the healing powers of your mind, you will be able to take back control of your fertility and influence it so that you become a mother.

I have clients who, during a hypnosis session with me, have gone back to the most simple, yet profound images. One remembered being a child watching a western where a woman was screaming repeatedly as she gave birth and died in extreme pain. That child said to herself 'I am *never* going to go through that.'

Another remembered being in her mother's arms as her mother described childbirth to her friends, saying, 'Oh, it was agony, I thought I was going to be ripped in half, and I thought I was dying from the pain. I bled non-stop and it went on for two days. It was brutal and horrendous.' That child had a similar thought-'I am *never* going to let that happen to *me*.'

I have witnessed clients who remember their own birth whilst in hypnosis. If it was very traumatic and frightening, it is the only experience of birth the subconscious has, and its job is to ensure that the person does not experience birth again, including giving birth herself. The subconscious mind is not logical. It's motivated by making sure you avoid anything that you link pain to, and only you can change this.

Baby Blocks

In over twenty-five years of working with women who are having difficulty conceiving, the same blocks come up over and over again. I have identified them here, and you may find you relate to one or more of them:

Block One: Fear of birth. This is one of the most common fears. So many women fear the unknown; they fear that the pain will be unbearable and unendurable, or, in extreme cases, that they or the baby may die. What they really fear is having no control. This fear can always be removed. Secondary infertility can often be caused by having had a problematic pregnancy or birth with the first baby.

Block Two: Fear of hospitals. If at any time, you or someone you know has had a bad experience in hospital, you might link being in a hospital to huge pain, and this can be strong enough to block conception.

Block Three: Fear of losing control of your body. We are taught in the West that we are happy when we are in control of ourselves and our bodies. This is actually not true, but the fear of losing that control may be dominant. It may not just be a fear of losing control of your body throughout pregnancy but a fear of not having the same body afterwards or ever again both internally and externally. A fear that you may not enjoy sex again, or that it may feel different and less pleasurable, is also very common.

Block Four: Guilt from a termination, miscarriage or stillbirth. Losing a baby is traumatic and overwhelming, and many women in this situation tell themselves, 'I can never go through this again.' This is a direct instruction to the mind to ensure you never *do* go through it again by never becoming pregnant again. When women have lost a baby at birth, they can feel terribly guilty that their body failed the baby. They have more guilt that having another child will make them forget the one they lost. Many women who terminate a pregnancy feel guilt and punish themselves at a subconscious level by denying themselves another baby, even though they are unaware that they are doing this. Their mind believes that being pregnant will bring up bad memories, so therefore pregnancy is best avoided.

Block Five: Fear of being a bad parent. This is another very common fear, especially if you had bad parents. We learn what we live. Your parents are the only role models you have, and society loves to tell us that we turn into our parents. However, many children of dysfunctional families go on to become much better parents. There is an abundance of parenting classes and many books, CDs, and DVDs on the market designed to help us become good and effective parents.

Block Six: Fear of losing your independence. This fear often affects career women. The fear of losing your social life, your freedom to travel, to be spontaneous, and the fear of losing financial independence and promotion can all be relevant, as can a fear of being trapped at home with a baby and feeling lonely, or of being unable to cope.

Block Seven: Fear of the baby. This block covers fears that the baby might scream all night, might be handicapped, might grow up to embarrass and shame you, might bankrupt you, might spoil or threaten your relationship with your partner.

Block Eight: Fear the baby will grow up and reject you. This fear particularly affects those who rejected their own parents or whose parents were estranged from, or had a poor relationship with, their own parents.

Block Nine: Fear of abandonment. The fear that your partner might leave you with the baby, if one of your parents did this, the fear will be more real.

Block Ten: Fear of the baby interfering in your relationship. Once the baby is born, you fear you can't be carefree and have sex whenever the mood takes you, or go out, or that your partner may become jealous of the attention you give to the baby or no longer find you sexy.

Block Eleven: Fear of not loving the baby. You fear that the baby might not like you, or you may not bond with it, or that your partner may prefer it over you and vice versa.

Block Twelve: Fear of age. A fear that you are too old to have a baby, too old to raise a baby, too set in your ways to enjoy a baby, and will be ridiculed around younger parents or mistaken for the grandparents.

"It is a trade secret but I will let you into it anyway, all healing is self healing."

Dr Albert Schweitzer.

STEP ONE:

Baby Steps

Changing Your Thoughts

- *Changing your thinking can change your life.*
- *Examples of how we can influence our fertility.*
- *Exercises demonstrating the power of thoughts.*

One of the most important steps in *Trying to get Pregnant (and Succeeding)* is Changing Your Thoughts. It is certainly the easiest to put into practice since it requires no financial outlay, and you do not need to devote long periods of time to it. As you begin to see how very easy it is to change your thinking, you will find this method creeping into other areas of your life, with wonderful results.

Thoughts are things, and all our thoughts have consequences. A thought is a cause, set in motion within us.

When it comes to conception and motherhood, our individual thoughts, beliefs, and expectations about pregnancy, birth, and babies will have a huge effect on our fertility, as our body is set up to mirror what is going on in our mind.

The strongest, most powerful force in the mind is its need to act in ways that match our thinking. The strongest force in the human personality is the need to remain consistent with how we define ourselves. In other words, your body responds to the pictures you make in your mind and constantly works to meet the picture. The subconscious mind has little capacity to reason, and believes whatever we tell it. Also, the subconscious mind has no sense of humour, so if you joke about being too reckless, too old, too tidy, too set in your ways to become a mother, your mind accepts this as a fact. You must stop thinking negative thoughts and using negative words (even in jest) if you want to have a baby.

You might be asking yourself, 'How can I stop thinking a thought, as it is instant?' It will get easier, I promise, and you can assist this by dismissing every negative thought you have and replacing it with a new, constructive one instead. Your thoughts belong to you, why would you keep them if you don't want them and don't want to believe them? Your thoughts are yours to change.

What we see, we become, and what we think about all the time, we become. People who are always ill think and talk about illness all the time.

I want you to think about expecting a baby and being an expectant mother. Keep your mind full of images of you as a mother-to-be. This is not the same as wishing you were pregnant. It sounds almost too simple, but it works. The power of thought may be simple, but thoughts themselves are enormously powerful and tremendously effective. You cannot have any thoughts and feelings without them being expressed in the body.

The way you are feeling about having a baby comes down to only two things: the pictures you make in your head and the words you are using. The mind responds to thoughts, words, and images that are symbolic. The good news is that you are able to choose the pictures you make in your mind and choose what you say, think, and feel about your fertility. A habit of thought precedes a habit of action, meaning if you believe you have to drink to relax, that belief will eventually become more powerful than the habit itself. This is why, when changing habits, you must also change the thoughts and beliefs related to them, thus ensuring that you don't return to them.

If you are undergoing any kind of fertility therapy, such as acupuncture, Chinese herbs, healing, or naturopathy, but doubting its ability to work, then these thoughts can and will work against the treatment you are having. However, if you believe that you will have a baby, and if you decide to change your thinking and also change some lifestyle habits, such as nutrition and vitamins, you will be much more likely to have a baby. This is particularly the case with IVF. Many women begin the IVF process focused on the 25 per cent success statistic and will not allow themselves to believe it will work for them on the first attempt, or at all. In fact, the 25 per cent statistic really only applies to the implantation of the embryos. The success rate of egg production and collection is frequently much higher than 25 per cent, and the fertilisation of the eggs is also higher than 25 per cent, even with ICSI. It has to be, or you could never get to the implantation process. At the most important stage-implanting the precious embryos-many women go into a state of fear and panic. They worry that the embryos are too fragile to stay in their womb, that they will fall out, that any jolt or movement will cause them to disintegrate. I have even known clients who've described their embryos as being like dandelion clocks about to fall apart at the slightest thing. In truth embryos are intelligent, and when they are in your womb you have the power to communicate with them, to harness that intelligence and to have them attach, implant, and grow securely in your womb. I always ask my clients to imagine their embryos as resilient, strong, robust, determined, and destined to be born with a powerful life force. My patients undergoing IVF learn to talk to the life force of their baby at every stage leading up to embryo transfer. They talk to the baby while they are taking the drugs to boost ovulation. They talk to it at the egg collection stage and again while they are in the clinic going through the procedure. They tell the embryo that in nine months they will be in another clinic delivering it as a healthy baby. They do this again at the fertilisation stage and at the embryo transfer. Then, at the happy stage when the embryo is back in their body, they talk to it and tell it how wanted and welcomed it is. They imagine their womb as being completely receptive and doing a perfect job of nourishing, nurturing, growing, and sustaining this new life throughout a perfect, happy pregnancy. They imagine the embryo knowing it is home, back where it's meant to be, inside its mother, growing perfectly until it is ready to be born.

In 2005, a forty-five-year-old Californian woman had a thirteen-year-old embryo implanted in her. This was one of the longest surviving embryos to date, and the mother, Debbie Beasley, had been told the chances of it working were minimal, not just because of the time the embryo was frozen but because the mother-to-be was forty-five and had suffered a near fatal allergic reaction to the fertility drugs, as well as having two miscarriages. Describing the moment of implantation, Mrs Beasley said, 'I put my hand over my abdomen and said, 'Welcome home, baby. She had been in this frozen place for so long, and I welcomed her into my warm womb and told her how much I wanted her.' Mrs Beasley went on to have a perfect baby daughter.

In May 2010 an American woman gave birth to a son after receiving a donated embryo that had been frozen for twenty years (the longest time an embryo has ever been frozen for). She also made a point of welcoming the embryo into her womb and seeing it as the baby's first home.

You probably plan to make your baby's first room really appealing and welcoming, with mobiles, toys, pretty wallpaper, and furnishings, but your baby's home for the first nine months is your body. It's your womb, and you can make it just as welcoming and receptive, and a good and happy place to be. Your womb has only one job to do throughout your life, and that is to prepare for and carry a baby, to sustain and nourish it, to nurture, protect, and grow it for nine months.

Your womb is an intelligent organ; it knows what to do and how to do it. It may sound silly to talk to your womb and to tell it to protect your baby to ensure that it implants, attaches, and sticks, and to nourish it and make sure it grows perfectly. However, you are talking to your womb anyway, every time you worry that the embryo won't make it or is too fragile to survive or that statistics are not on your side. When you talk to your womb and embryo, you are doing something powerful, because every thought you think has a physical reaction in your body, and your body *has to* react and respond in a way that matches your thinking.

Because of the mind's ability to believe and accept without question, to take on as an absolute fact all our thoughts and dialogue, including the internal dialogue or self-talk that goes on inside our heads, it follows that if you constantly tell yourself you might lose your baby, or if you refuse to get your hopes up in case you are disappointed, you are more likely to have that very thing happen. However, if you keep telling yourself its working because you and your baby have such a powerful connection that is both physical and emotional, you are more likely to receive *that* outcome.

Babies in the womb have been proven to react with distress to loud sounds and new-born babies recognise their mother's voice and heartbeat. Your baby will hear you when you talk to it, so tell it how much it is wanted and how much faith you have that it will grow and develop perfectly until that wonderful moment when it is ready to be born to you.

Tell your baby to grow healthy, strong bones, perfect organs, and a robust heart. Show it how to develop by looking at pictures of developing foetuses, imagining your baby at each stage, and telling it at each stage to grow exactly as the foetus in the picture is doing. I show my patients pictures and diagrams of the embryo and foetus so they know what it looks like. My favourite book for incredible pictures of developing babies in the womb is *Life* by Lennart Nilsson, and my website **www.tryingtogetpregnant.co.uk** has pictures showing you the stages of a developing baby. You can use these images to talk to your baby about what it is doing at each stage.

When I was visiting the museum at Bart's Hospital, I was so moved by how perfect the foetuses on display were that I wanted to take one home, to show to my patients that they were miracles. There was, on display in a bell jar, a fallopian tube containing a foetus from an ectopic pregnancy. The baby was the size of a small tomato but its features were perfect. There were twins floating in another bell jar that were the size of chipolatas, but again their features were so perfect. One had its mouth open, and I could even see its tiny perfect tongue.

These are the images you need to keep in your mind throughout conception and throughout your pregnancy. See a perfect, happy, healthy, wanted baby growing perfectly in your body and your body doing everything it needs to do to sustain and grow your baby. You and your baby are a perfect team, working together and communicating with each other all the time.

Your body loves and nourishes your baby throughout your pregnancy. It knows what to do and it does it. Your baby also knows what to do, and is growing and developing on target, perfectly.

Your baby will respond to your words and thoughts. Buying a few items in advance of its arrival is a mark of your faith that it will be born, while buying nothing is a mark of your fear that it may not arrive. Fear stands for *False Expectations Appearing Real*. Worry is a sustained form of imagining what you don't want to happen, until your body reacts as if it is happening anyway, because your mind cannot tell the difference between what is real and what is imagined.

When people do not allow themselves to believe something will work, just in case it doesn't, it never stops them from mourning its failure. If you embark on a pregnancy telling yourself it may not go to full term, and then it doesn't, your distress will not be any less. It's much better to tell yourself it will work, and to see it working, than to plan for failure and to allow for disappointment. You cannot minimise disappointment by planning and preparing for it in advance, so it's much healthier not to expect disappointment.

I have met patients who dread going to the bathroom after embryo transfer because they fear finding some blood-proof it has not worked. Expecting this and focusing on it in advance is detrimental to the success of your pregnancy. If you tell yourself you are forgetful or clumsy, you will become that way, and even telling this to young children can cause them to act and become clumsy and forgetful. You must abandon negative thoughts about your ability to have a baby immediately. Don't even entertain the idea or put words or pictures relating to it in your mind.

Trying to get Pregnant (and Succeeding)

Some doctors believe that when migraines, depression, or period pains run in families, it is because the mind has accepted this as inevitable, and the body acts accordingly. Often, when working with clients, they say things like, 'Everyone in my family has miscarried,' or 'All the women in my family have had problems conceiving,' or 'My mother suffered terribly with problem pregnancies, and I'm just like her,' and so on, without being aware of how they are identifying with the symptom.

Studies have been done that show that spontaneous miscarriages occur more frequently if the baby does not feel wanted.[6] This has much to do with your baby's developed hearing and its connection to your thoughts. If you knew for a fact that your baby was tuned in to you and heard your words and picked up your thoughts, you would make more of an effort to be positive about its presence in your body and in your life. The truth is, your baby *is* tuned in to you 24/7.

In some tribes, pregnant women wear a pink ribbon around their neck from the moment they are aware they are pregnant. This tells others to respect their pregnancy and not to shout around them or indulge in negative talk, as they know the developing baby is pure sensation, and they respect and honour this. We need to do the same.

When I was carrying my daughter, I talked to her all the time, and when I told her to kick for me, she did. I was told twice in my pregnancy that I was losing her. Of course I panicked and was fearful, but I lay down and stroked my stomach, told her how much I loved and wanted her. I told her to stay with me. I told her no baby in the world was more wanted and loved than she was. I told her how much her daddy and her grandparents wanted her, and I asked her to stay. It made me feel so much better than feeling helpless and waiting for a miscarriage. I had

---

6 Thomas Verney The Secret Life of the Unborn Child
New Scientist magazine 11/03/2010
Dr Kazuyuki Shinorhara Nagasaki university Japan

negative thoughts in my pregnancy, but I counteracted them and apologised to my baby whenever I said or did something negative. All pregnant mothers have had the experience of talking to their baby and the baby kicking in response, so we all know that babies respond to our words and thoughts. So do embryos, and so do foetuses- why wouldn't they?

When we long for that feeling of lying on the beach, absorbing the warmth of the sun, hearing the waves lapping, feeling the warm water, it's because that is a foetal memory. People love the beach and find the warmth and the sound of the water relaxing because it reminds them of being in the womb. We mostly sleep in the foetal position, again because it's a foetal memory. If we can remember being in the womb years and years later, we must have senses that are active while we are there. This knowledge will help you communicate with your baby, knowing it is responding.

On one occasion, I was doing hypnotic regression with a man who hated any loud noise and reacted very badly to it, which made his life extremely limited. Under hypnosis, he relived a scene in which he was hiding in a cupboard and could hear drums that were so loud, he felt sick. Suddenly he said, 'No, I'm not in a cupboard. I'm in my mother's womb, and she's hiding in a cupboard, and it's her heartbeat that is so loud, it's making me really distressed.' Later he asked his mother if this could have been true, and she said when she was seven months pregnant and living in Kenya, the house was burgled whilst she was alone in it, and she hid in a cupboard fearing for her life.

Another of my clients was brought to her session by her father, as she could not go anywhere alone because she was severely claustrophobic. While I was regressing her back to the cause of the claustrophobia, she went back to her own breech birth. Her shoulders were stuck. She was traumatised and felt trapped. Her father confirmed that this was a true description of her birth, although she had not known that before she came to see me.

Another client who went through life feeling and re-experiencing loss many times over, talked to her mother about the work we were doing and how I had identified that she was very focused on loss. Her mother then told her that she was an identical twin, but her sister was miscarried during the pregnancy. At some level she knew this; she even remembered the loss she felt when her sister was no longer sharing a womb with her.

A mother of one-year-old twins in London reported that her children's favourite activity was holding the shower curtain over each other and kissing and touching each other through it every time they were in the bath. She was convinced they were replaying an activity they had carried out in the womb.

The body must match what is going on in the mind; it is never the other way around. The mind won't match what is going on in the body, because the thought always has to come first, and every thought is eventually expressed in the body or through the body. The way you feel about your ability to have a baby, can become an expectation that you live up to in your mind, and then in your body. Your feelings about parenthood and the beliefs you hold about pregnancy and birth are having an enormous effect on you right now. Thoughts and beliefs affect us greatly, and your thoughts about being a parent are affecting your body this very second. The body mimics the mind's thoughts. Every thought we have creates a physical reaction in the body and an emotional response, but our thoughts and beliefs are not fixed, and are ours to change. Thinking positive, powerful thoughts and telling yourself your reproductive system is young and super-fertile causes it to respond and behave in a way that matches those thoughts. Whereas telling yourself that your body is old, dried up, and without any useful eggs has the opposite effect. Our cells listen and respond to our thinking.

Changing our thinking does not always happen automatically. Sometimes we have to keep at it because we are becoming conditioned to believe infertility is a curse that over 25 per cent of us will encounter. That is not true all over the world, and it does not have to be true for you, even if you have been diagnosed with it. Our thoughts are so instant; it is easy to feel that they are controlling us. But instead we must think: Where did that belief come from? Who put it there? Why am I choosing to believe this? You might have to work at it initially, but it will become second nature after a while, and it will be worth it.

Everything we do and everything we want is because of how it makes us feel or will make us feel. We want to have a baby because we believe this will make our lives better. Believing you will make it happen, and seeing it happen in your mind, will cause you to feel better physically, mentally, and emotionally.

Since our body doesn't age in the way we have been led to believe, it is not true that you only have a 2 per cent chance of conceiving after the age of forty. When I was forty-four, I was having a smear test, and the doctor asked me what method of contraception I used. I told him that since my partner was working abroad and I only saw him on weekends, I didn't use any. He was shocked and said, 'Look, you must be careful. We see this all the time women in their forties who think they won't get pregnant, and then they do. You are taking a big risk.' Yet women who go to the doctor and say, 'I am forty-five and I really want to have a baby' are told they have a 2 per cent chance of it happening.

After teenagers, the next highest rate of abortions are carried out on women who are in their forties who thought they could not conceive, abandoned birth control, and became pregnant. The number of women giving birth in their forties has increased by 70 per cent in the last ten years, and the rate of women having terminations in their forties has increased by a third in less than ten years.[7] In 2010, there were 27,731 births in Britain to women over forty. As it happens, I got pregnant accidently when I was forty-seven. I am convinced it was because I spent so much time telling clients they are super fertile. I lost the baby, but that had nothing to do with my age, it was an issue to do with the father's genes. After I lost the baby, my consultant told me to be really careful, as he was worried I would get pregnant again, and because my partner had a defective gene, it was not advisable.

When I was at school, we were counselled against the dangers of heavy petting and warned that even without ejaculation (in fact, even without penetration) women have become pregnant, as a rogue sperm can be released in pre-ejaculate and can swim into the vagina, and impregnation can occur. Yet I have had women in tears in my office because they have been told that their husband only has sixty million sperm, and it isn't enough to impregnate them. The average ejaculate contains about three hundred million, but only about two hundred of these sperm will get close enough to the egg to fertilise it. You don't need anywhere near three hundred million.

You only need one sperm to conceive your baby. The two hundred sperm that get close to the egg are useful,

---

[7] The figures on older childbirth released by the Office for National Statistics said that 27,731 UK mothers older than 40 gave birth in 2010 a 70% increase since 2001.
Royal College of Midwives Number-of babies-born-to mothers-over 40-TRIPLED-in a decade
Department of health abortion statistics for 2010 show numbers have risen by a third in women over 40
Office for national statistics 30% increase in terminations of women over 40.

as some of them will bash against the shell and weaken it, but just one sperm will break through and fertilise your egg. You have the power to influence that one perfect sperm to swim to and fertilise your egg. Your egg gives off a powerful chemical in the fluid to draw the correct sperm to it. Imagine this chemical as super-powerful and the sperm as a scud missile directed by the chemical to a perfect result of fertilisation, conception, and impregnation. Once the sperm are in your body, you can influence them, as they are now yours, so imagine the sperm like a heat-seeking missile being pulled towards the egg and doing its job like an elite special forces operative.

I work with many fathers-to-be, and I tell them to imagine their sperm as super swimmers-the Mark Spitz or Michael Phelps of sperm. They imagine a special squad of two hundred sperm, like super elite corps, the SAS of sperm, doing a perfect job of fertilisation. If they have been told they don't have enough sperm or have poor quality sperm, then we imagine the sperm increasing in quality and quantity, since the body changes all the time. Sperm, like blood, can be of poor quality but can dramatically improve. When a man has sex with a regular partner, he ejaculates half the amount of sperm as he does when he has sex with a new lover. A man will ejaculate more than six hundred million sperm with a new lover and three hundred million sperm with a long-standing partner. This is because nature has determined that the species must go on, so doubling sperm outtake with a new partner is more likely to ensure a pregnancy. The same thing happens with animals. The male can go on having sex every time a new female is introduced to him, but he cannot go on having sex with the same female. If a captive rat is constantly introduced to new females, he will literally fornicate until he drops dead. So will rams and many other animals. Before this infuriates you, be aware that women do something similar. When a woman has sex with a new lover, her cervix tilts to attract sperm and encourage pregnancy. If you have been with the same partner for years and have not become pregnant, try meeting in a hotel as strangers, dress up as a traffic warden, nurse, waitress, stripper, air hostess, business woman, whatever it takes, and ask your partner to dress up and role play as a stranger, too. He can be a doctor, pilot, soldier, builder, whatever appeals to you. Have sex without talking much, and imagine you are with a stranger, as this may double your chances of conception. (Some of my client's stories of how they conceived in this way are hilarious.)

The average male produces seventy-two million sperm daily, and with every ejaculation a man loses between two hundred and six hundred million sperm, so having sex too often can use up his good sperm. Ideally, you should have sex every other day around the time of planned conception, so you have sperm in your womb but don't allow your partner to run out of good-quality sperm. Have sex every other day, four days before and four days after ovulation. Sperm will live for between two and five days inside a woman and can last even longer, especially if you imagine them doing so.

Intrauterine insemination (IUI) is the process whereby sperm is collected and placed back into the woman's uterus as high as possible so it's closer to the egg, making conception more likely, as the sperm are already near the egg and don't have to swim far. Men love rear entry sex because it is so deep, although some women find it uncomfortable because it's too deep. The closer the sperm can be deposited to the woman's cervix, the better the chances of conception, so choose positions that allow for the deepest possible penetration. Think of doggy style as DIY IUI. Having your partner ejaculate in the rear entry position (doggy style) is the most effective method for conception, as just like IUI, the sperm are deposited much nearer to the egg, so it has the energy to break through the shell and fertilise it. It's helpful to imagine this as your partner ejaculates while you are having sex. It can take sperm up to five hours to reach the egg, although usually it takes the sperm between five minutes and one hour. It's been proven that if the woman orgasms during sex, the contractions help move the sperm upwards and into the cervix, so try to avoid clinical sex (where you are doing it just to conceive), and remember that you are more likely to conceive if you relax.

If you change negative beliefs, you can change your biochemistry. Just because we have held something to be true for a number of years, this is not a good enough reason to hold on to it forever. Remember, you used to believe in Santa Claus once and then changed your beliefs as you acquired new information. When we control our thoughts, anything is possible. If we believe that we are fat or unlovable, we begin to manifest the thoughts we are holding, until we eventually become a living, walking, talking expression of them. A belief or feeling that we are unlovable is the common denominator of most of the emotional problems in the Western world. Many women cannot conceive because they fear they won't be good enough parents, especially if they did not have good enough parents themselves.

The power of thought alone can change the physical body and affect our mental health and our immune system. What we think is possible affects our body. People have been observed to get drunk on alcohol-free beverages because they think they are potent, or high on nothing but their thoughts or beliefs about the substance they are ingesting. This thought process can become even stronger when it occurs in groups, and mass sickness can occur on airlines or at functions and at receptions. The same thing can happen in crowds, leading to mass hysteria or anger.

At the Monterey Park football stadium in Los Angeles, several people became ill during a game, with symptoms of food poisoning. The on-site doctor treating them discovered that they had all consumed fizzy drinks from the vending machines at the stadium. He decided that fermentation or contamination may have taken place within the machines, and eager that no one else be put at risk, he put out an announcement telling people not to use the vending machines and described the symptoms over the tannoy. Almost at once, the stadium became a sea of people retching and fainting, including many who had not drunk anything from the suspected machines. Five ambulances carried people back and forth between the hospital and stadium before it was discovered that the vending machines were safe, and the illness of the first group was unrelated. You can find examples everywhere of the power of thought, suggestion and beliefs.

Thoughts have very direct consequences. At Massachusetts General Hospital, anaesthesiologist Dr Henry Beecher found that 30 per cent of a drug's or a doctor's success is due to the patient's expectation of a desired outcome, or the "placebo effect." The American Society of Psychosomatic Medicine founded in 1955 further explored the placebo effect.[8] Today drug companies routinely discard over 30 per cent of drug test results, because if a person believes a drug to be effective, it can have more effect on him than the drug itself. This is why many repeat drug prescriptions are placebos and why whenever a drug is tested it must also be tested on a control group who think they are receiving the same drug but are in fact receiving a placebo.

Our beliefs about the drugs and medicines we take can be even more significant in our recovery than the pharmaceutical components of the drugs themselves. Dr Beecher became famous for doing extensive research and numerous studies that concluded that while we may believe a particular drug has healed or cured us, in fact

---

8 Beecher, H.K., Research and the Individual: Human Studies, Little, Brown, (Boston), 1970.

our belief system was the real healing force. In his 1955 paper *The Powerful Placebo* Dr Beecher went on record stating: *"A drug's usefulness is a direct result of not only the chemical properties of the drug, but also the patient's belief in the usefulness and effectiveness of the drug."*

In America, when a new drug, which was formulated to re-grow hair, was tested, the group given placebo pills re-grew hair, despite many of them having been bald for years. In another test in England, a group believing they were receiving a new form of chemotherapy lost all their hair purely because they expected to, since unbeknownst to them they were receiving placebos.

Our brain converts our expectations into chemical realities. Thoughts are things, and thoughts always have an effect on our bodies. Thinking about hunger, sex, or tiredness will cause us to generate feelings and physical reactions, linked to our thinking. Reading books that describe immense cold can make us shiver and grow goose bumps, while watching a scary or emotional film can generate feelings of fear or emotion within ourselves that seem quite real.

Of course advertising companies know all about this and use it to their advantage. Images of food can cause us to feel hungry, while images of drinks make us thirsty. Even very young children have been proven to respond to adverts. In fact one of the reasons the children's television programme *Sesame Street* was devised was to maximise young children's ability to respond to television adverts. The same successful format, short bursts of message, sound, and colour used to make adverts, were used to make that programme.

We see more examples of the power of thought in telepathy, and in people who appear to have unusual powers, such as faith healers and mind readers. I believe in faith healing, but I also believe that just being around someone we perceive as powerful, or being in a place like Lourdes can have such a powerful effect on the belief system that we can see results regardless of what is real and what is imagined.

Years ago a client came to see me because he wanted to stop drinking. He sat on the other side of my desk while I asked him some questions, and suddenly he looked at me and said, 'I can't answer any more questions, this hypnosis is too powerful,' and he slumped back in his chair, closed his eyes, and went into a trance purely because he expected to. In fact I had not hypnotised him.

As he was already responding to his own power of thought, I used the situation to convince his subconscious that he would not drink again and to uncover the causes of drinking and the beliefs that made him drink too much. He called me some weeks later to tell me how thrilled he was that he no longer wanted to drink, and to this day, I have clients who come in after being referred by this man. They always tell me that he is a major fan of hypnosis, and of me, because I had such a powerful effect on him. I didn't ever have the heart to tell him that I did very little. His own belief system stopped him from drinking.

Further examples of this can be seen in people from other cultures who think they have been cursed, and then develop symptoms linked to their beliefs and sometimes even die. In Africa this is known as 'shaking' or 'pointing the bone.' If the witch doctor 'shakes the bone,' the recipient of the curse will expect to get ill and perhaps die. Even in cases where medical intervention has taken place to cure the resulting illness or symptoms, it hasn't always been enough to overcome that person's belief system, which thinks 'I am cursed and dying.' The belief system is the stronger force and has more power than anything else.

People who have moved to places like Haiti and scorn the belief in voodoo and similar traditions, often come to see something in it, because it is all around them. They become somewhat influenced by the pervasive effect it has on them. Other common examples occur with the symptoms of phantom pregnancies and psychosomatic illnesses.

A thought is a cause set in motion within us. The Bible says, '*As a man thinketh in his heart, so is he.*'

Dr Ellen Langer, a psychologist at Harvard Medical School, put this to the test in 1979, when she took a group of men, all over seventy-five years old, to a retreat in the country for seven days. Prior to leaving, the group was put through a series of tests to establish each person's biological age. Among other things, they were tested for hearing, vision, grip, finger length, muscle mass, bone density, perception, physical strength, blood, hormones, and so on. The retreat had been designed to recreate the year 1959, and the participants even wore badges with pictures of themselves from twenty years ago. They watched films, sitcoms, and newsreels, and listened to music of the 50's. All the magazines and newspapers were from the 50's, and the participants were not allowed to bring with them anything from a later date.

The group then purposefully pretended it was twenty years ago. The conversation and everything else going on around them was deliberately engineered to enable and encourage each man to act as he had when he was fifty-five rather than seventy-five, while a control group went to the same retreat but did not have to pretend or live in the artificially backdated environment.

By willingly participating and living this experiment, the main participants were subconsciously tricking themselves, and consequently their cells, to believe they were younger. During and at the end of the seven days, they were put through the same tests again...and all had reversed their age by a minimum of seven years. Some had reversed their age by over ten years. By contrast, the control group improved very marginally in a few areas but declined in others.

Trying to get Pregnant (and Succeeding)

In 2010, the BBC recruited Dr Ellen Langer to repeat the programme with a group of British celebrities. Those taking part included the actresses Liz Smith who was eighty-eight years old, and Sylvia Syms, seventy-six; cricket umpire Dickie Bird, seventy-seven; dancer Lionel Blair, seventy-seven; and journalist Derek Jameson, eighty. Just as in the 1979 experiment, the group stayed in a large country house that had been fitted with furnishings and kitchen and electrical appliances that would have been seen in 1975. The newspapers and television programmes available to them were from 1975, and each person's bedroom was decorated to look as much like it would have in the 70's, complete with personal mementoes from the time.

The experiment started off like the earlier American one, and the participants had to take care of themselves right from the beginning. When they arrived at the house where they would be staying for a week, they had to carry their own bags upstairs. Liz Smith was the only one who didn't do it, as she had been assigned to a bedroom on the ground floor. She was unable to walk more than a few steps without the aid of two sticks and had to use a wheelchair when going outside. Within days, each of the celebrities had considerably improved. Liz Smith managed to walk around the kitchen with just one stick. She even managed a bit of dancing! Sylvia Syms ran around the garden with two dogs, with youthful gusto. They all showed great improvements just halfway through the week.

Then some professional carers came in and offered to do everything for the participants. Some agreed and quickly reverted to their old selves. When the carers left again, in the afternoon, things soon got back on track. After the help left, Lionel Blair said it had made him feel much older. Liz Smith agreed. Sylvia Syms had steadfastly refused any help.

Baby Steps

By the end of the seven days, it was clear that all of participants were much better at doing various things than they had been just one week earlier. They all had better balance, flexibility, upper and lower body strength, and a more positive outlook on life. Liz Smith was able to walk more than 140 paces across the garden, with only one stick. In the final physical examination, she was able to stand on one leg without holding on to anything. She even went out dancing when she returned home! Lionel Blair danced with a tap dancing group and looked very agile, matching the movements and speed of the men who were about one-third his age. Sylvia Syms is now helping with a charity that assists older people. She said that when she first started on the experiment, she was in considerable pain all the time from back injuries, and she had no energy. She was running about by the end of the exercise, and said she had no back pain and had more energy. Derek Jameson could hardly get up the stairs at the beginning, but halfway through, he was doing step-ups on a low step. At the start, he couldn't even put his own socks on, so bad was his flexibility, but by the end, he could do it. Dickie Bird felt as if he had a new lease on life. His strength, memory, and agility improved. Since suffering a stroke, he had been living without much contact with other people and had lost a lot of confidence, but was determined to take part in life again. It was particularly satisfying to see him laughing and enjoying himself, as since retirement he had become a self-confessed recluse. As Jameson was packing to go home at the end of the week, he explained what had happened to make them all feel so much younger. He said that he'd forgotten that he was eighty, that he did slip back into the 1970s and lived in that world of thirty-five years ago.

These experiments proved that what you believe is so important in determining how you age, and what happens if you think you are too old to conceive. If you think and act old, you may grow old prematurely, whereas if you think and act younger, you can remain younger physically, mentally, and biologically.

In another BBC programme, members of the public were asked to make sentences out of words to test their language proficiency. The first group was given words that are usually associated with old age, such as 'obedient,' 'accepting,' 'wise,' 'courteous,' 'alone,' 'sentimental,' and 'careful.' The group were filmed entering the building, and again after the test, as they left the room and walked along a corridor. Most of them walked more slowly (some ten or twenty per cent slower) as if using words associated with old age had made them behave older.

A second group participated in the same test but used words usually associated with youth, such as 'ambition,' 'freedom,' 'attractive,' 'fashion,' and 'passion.' Most of them walked more quickly afterwards-as much as ten or fifteen per cent faster.

In another experiment, people were told they were going to be tested to see if they would be good fighter pilots. They wore pilot overalls and were tested in a flight simulator of a Harrier jump jet. Their eyesight was tested before and afterwards. Most of them could read more letters on the eye chart after the experiment. Their eyes hadn't improved, but it is thought their brains were working harder-as if they were still trying to be like fighter pilots. Fighter pilots need excellent vision, so their brains were trying to give them that.

Changing our thinking and our behaviour has a physical effect on the ageing of our minds and bodies. Since these tests proved that we can become biologically seven years younger, and more, in just seven days, we can learn a lot from them.

You can do the same thing. You can become biologically and physically younger by changing your beliefs and recreating your notion of who you are and what you associate with pregnancy and motherhood. Changing your focus and your language can improve and boost your fertility. Incidentally, thoughts always affect the skin, which is why it boasts a rosy glow when we are in love or feeling happy and good about ourselves, and looks grey or drawn when we are grieving or deeply unhappy.[9]

So...change your thoughts about your ability to have a perfect pregnancy and a perfect baby, and delete all negative words connected to motherhood from your vocabulary. Thoughts even affect our immune system. By changing your language and by making some modifications in the way you eat, sleep, and behave, you can greatly influence your fertility. It all starts with adjusting how you think. Everything that is going on in your body, including how you react to being pregnant, has to start with the mind. For any area of your life that you want to change or control, you must begin by transforming your thoughts.

Thoughts control feelings.
Feelings control actions.
Actions control events.

I don't really like the word 'control,' and I try to avoid using it, but there are certain areas like health and pregnancy where it is essential that we take control of our health. In life, so many things appear to be out of our control, but in fact the only real control we have over events is what we choose to think of them, what we decide something means, because the way we interpret an event or the meaning we attach to an event, will affect us more than the event itself.

---

[9] When you're happy all your feel good chemicals are moving through your veins, and this increases the circulation to the skin on your face.

Baby Exercises: 1.

Since you will believe it when you see it, I am going to show you how every thought you think has a physical effect and an emotional response within your body. I would like you to do a few very simple and perfectly safe exercises to demonstrate the amazing physical powers of thought so that you can feel it and experience it for yourself rather than just read about it.

Stand up, with your feet slightly apart. Close your eyes, and begin to imagine that just behind you there is a huge magnet, pulling you and rocking you backwards. Really focus on the magnet. See it as a huge U shape, with the red paint on the ends, just behind your shoulder blades.

You will almost immediately feel yourself swaying and rocking and tipping backwards. You might even notice that your knees lock and your toes come off the floor.

Now imagine the magnet has moved to just under your chin pulling you forwards. Again, as you think about the magnet pulling you forwards, your own power of thought will cause you to rock forwards, to sway forwards and to move off your heels.

Now imagine the magnet has moved to your right shoulder and notice your body swaying in that direction; then imagine it moving to the left. The more you focus on the magnet, the stronger the pull will become. Just notice it happening.

If you prefer, you can close your eyes and ask a friend to describe a magnet behind you, then in front of you, and then at either side of your shoulder, or ask someone to read this section to you.

Of course there is no magnet there, but you are beginning to see and feel for yourself your mind's ability to accept whatever you tell it, whether it's based on fact or fiction. As your mind accepts the thought of the magnet, it then works to have you react to it, even though it only exists in your imagination.

The same is true with every thought that you have. If you think of having a baby, your mind has to accept that and work on it, and even more importantly, your cells and your immune system react to the thought. If you think of being infertile, the same thing happens, so one thought can generate positive reactions and another thought will generate negative reactions within the body. Whether these thoughts are based on fact or fiction is irrelevant to the mind, because it cannot tell the difference.

Here is another safe and simple exercise to prove to you that thought really is the most powerful thing. You can do this while sitting or standing.

Close your eyes. Stretch both hands out in front of you at shoulder height, and close both hands as if you are holding reins or a bar in each hand. Now begin to imagine that in your left hand you are holding an enormous red fire bucket filled with about forty pounds of heavy wet sand. Feel the weight of that bucket in your fingers. Feel the weight moving up to your wrist, your elbow, and now your shoulder. Feel it getting heavier and heavier by the second, and notice that your arm is being pulled down by the weight of the bucket. The more you focus on the bucket, on its colour and size and contents, the heavier your arm is becoming, and the more it is being drawn downwards.

As your left arm continues moving downwards, imagine that you are holding in your right hand the biggest helium-filled balloon. See the balloon's colour as bright blue. See it as almost bigger than you are. Feel the string in your hand. As helium is lighter than air, and because this balloon is firmly held in your right hand, you will notice that your right arm is moving upwards, travelling up higher and higher, becoming lighter and lighter, almost floating upwards of its own accord. As you think about the balloon and bucket, notice the difference in your arms. One is heavy, one is light, one is moving up the other is moving down. The cause of this is your thought process. You may prefer to memorise this or to have someone read this part to you, as you keep your eyes shut. Again the point is to show you how easy it is to influence your mind, and to prove to you that thoughts have a very real effect on our bodies.

Thoughts affect chemical changes in the body. Positive thinking can produce chemicals in the brain and cells of the central nervous system, which then affect the immune system. This can then produce natural killer cells (NKs), T-cells, and white blood cells, which can destroy certain types of illness and fight bacteria and viruses. Because the strongest force in the mind is its need to make us act in ways that match our thinking, it is vital to change any negative thoughts and expectations connected to fertility and pregnancy.

If you want to have a healthy pregnancy and a healthy baby, you must *focus on how you want to be, never on how you don't want to be.*

In other words:

Keep your mind on what you want and off what you don't want. Focus only on what you want to move towards and accomplish, never on the opposite, which is what you want to leave behind.

This becomes easier as you find the flip side of every negative thought and use that instead.

Whatever we focus on, we move towards. Whatever we focus on, we experience and feel. Whatever we focus on, we get more of, as it becomes more real to us.

If you focus on having an injection or the pressure in your ears during a flight descent, you can make it painful, but if you focus on something else, you may not even notice the sensations.

Now, using a notebook, write down all your thoughts about pregnancy, babies, and motherhood. Write out every negative thought that you have been led to believe about having a baby, on one page, and write out new, more appropriate thoughts on the opposite page. Keep on writing until you have run out of thoughts, but don't be surprised if more come to you later (As they do, write them down, too). The reason I want you to write down your negative thoughts is because often we are not even aware of our thoughts. We hold them, we act on them, but we don't confront them or look at them or think, is this relevant to me, has it ever been relevant to me?

We update our hairstyles, our makeup and our homes, yet fail to update our thinking. Before we can change our thinking, we need to identify and discover our thoughts. We have to become more aware of our thoughts, in order to update them, and to review and revise them.

Take some time to uncover your thoughts about your fertility, and become more and more aware of how you think. Find and root out any negative thoughts, confront them, change them, eliminate and eradicate them. As you start writing, your thoughts will begin to flow from you. At this stage don't stop to analyse them, just keep on writing. It doesn't matter if you write reams, or just a few thoughts, as long as they are *your* thoughts.

This programme will allow you to end your old, negative thinking, and in its place, you will have new, powerful, positive thoughts that you really believe in, and which will affect your biology in a more favourable way.

Here are some examples to get you started on the process of changing your thinking.

Examples of Negative Thinking:

- Nature doesn't expect us to have babies after thirty-five.
- My eggs diminish in quantity and quality after thirty-five.
- I am much more likely to have a handicapped baby or a miscarriage at my age.

- I will look stupid in the clinic and at my child's school, as I will be older than all the other mothers. I might even be mistaken for a grandparent.
- I don't know how to raise a baby I might not be able to cope.
- I won't be able to function without sleep.
- I can't afford to take time of work and I'm not sure I will ever be able to afford a baby.

New Thoughts:

- Humans are living longer, and today forty-five is more like thirty-five, and thirty-five is more like twenty-five. Thousands of women have babies after thirty-five.
- I have a young healthy body, and I will be a healthy parent.
- My eggs are young, grade-A, superior eggs. I have all the eggs I need, and the most perfect, resilient egg will become my child.
- Since a perfect egg is being fertilised by my partner's perfect sperm, it will become a perfect, healthy baby in a perfect, full-term pregnancy.
- I will learn how to raise my baby and cope perfectly well like other new mothers and I will use all the help available to me.
- I will get enough sleep as I can sleep when my baby sleeps and babies sleep a lot.
- I will be a wonderful parent, with time, love, and patience for my child. I will find a way of doing my job, having my baby and managing financially.

Baby Steps

Today you have learnt the absolute power of thoughts and how to change your thinking. You know that thoughts are things and that every single thought you have has a physical effect on your body and an emotional effect on your mind. All your thoughts have consequences; your healthy thoughts have healthy consequences, while negative thoughts will eventually have negative consequences.

All thoughts in the mind produce responses in the body, so by applying the techniques in this book and learning to only accept positive thoughts about conception, you can programme your body to conceive, carry, and deliver your perfect child.

You have learnt that your thoughts are yours to change, update, review, and remove, as they cease to be appropriate for you. You have also proved to yourself, with the physical exercises, the power of your thoughts on your body, and this will give you the proof and incentive you need to take control of your thoughts rather than let them control you.

"Man is what he believes."

Anton Chekhov.

STEP TWO:

Misconceptions

*You won't believe it when you see it.
You will see it when you believe it.
What we see and believe, we
become.*

In Step one you looked at your thinking. Now, in Step two, it is time to work on your beliefs. Aren't thoughts and beliefs the same thing? Well, no, they are not quite the same thing. Many people think one thing and believe another, so their mind is in a form of conflict. It is very important that your thoughts and beliefs be congruent, that they match and go together, so that they complement each other, especially if you want to have a baby.

Imagine thinking that you want a baby, while believing that you might be an awful mother or that your husband might love the baby more than he loves you. Or thinking that you would love to get pregnant whilst believing that pregnancy is scary and hospitals are even scarier. If you can imagine that, then you understand how thoughts and beliefs differ, and can conflict with each other. A thought is something we hold in our minds, that we shape and form in our brain, using language and pictures, whereas beliefs can be so silent yet immediate that we are not always aware they are there, yet they are absolutely influencing us.

For instance, if you believe that you are scared of cats or bees, your body will react to that belief as soon as you see a cat or a bee, without you thinking about it at all. Your belief will set off an immediate reaction of fear within your body, which may respond by having palpitations, shaking, sweating, and even feeling sick. Your thoughts may be busy saying, 'It's only a little cat. It can't harm me. It's far away. It's more scared of me,' but your thoughts alone are having little or no impact on your belief. And so it is with our beliefs on fertility. We may not be aware of them, but we react to them very strongly, and they are influencing us twenty-four hours a day. We can change our thoughts quite easily with practice and repetition, but beliefs can take a little longer. The way to change a belief is to introduce doubt…to question the belief.

If you have beliefs you want to change, start questioning where they originated from and why you are holding them, and then begin to introduce doubt to their validity. As soon as you question a belief, you are voicing doubt and no longer fully hold that belief to be true. The more you question a belief, the more you doubt it. This programme will enable you to doubt and question much that you have been taught about fertility. As you doubt your old beliefs, your mind will be receptive and open to accept new beliefs that will have a much more beneficial effect on your ability to have your baby.

Misconceptions

It can sometimes only take seconds for a belief to change. Look at the example of historic runner, Roger Bannister. It had been accepted and believed since records began, that a human could not run a mile in under four minutes. Bannister was determined to change this, and he began by changing his own belief system. First, he saw the four minutes as 240 seconds, and then repeatedly visualised himself running a mile in 239 seconds. He used a form of self-hypnosis and visualisation to do this, and changed the general belief system about the mile. Within one year, thirty-seven more people ran a mile in under four minutes, followed by three hundred runners the following year.

There are examples all around us of people who have held a belief to be true for years, and then overnight their belief system changed. People might discover that a partner has been unfaithful or that their father is not their biological parent. More positively, people who are told they can't have children become pregnant, and people who don't believe in God change their belief immediately and permanently when something miraculous happens. We used to believe the earth was flat, and that if you picked up a baby too much you would spoil it. We have since learned that these things are not true.

A whole generation of babies were brought up on beliefs outlined by a leading childcare expert of the time, Dr Benjamin Spock. Spock later decided that he was wrong and publicly denounced his own beliefs on national television, apologising to a generation of mothers and advising them to disregard everything he had taught them. Many of these mothers had overridden their own nurturing instincts to kiss or pick up their infants because Dr Spock told them not to, and they believed he must be right. After all, he was a child authority, so they believed him.

As with thoughts, our beliefs are ours to change. Even definite, rigid beliefs can be changed. You have nothing to lose and everything to gain by deciding to continually assess and review your beliefs and to only hold beliefs about babies, birth, and motherhood that will benefit you and empower you.

There are different types and intensities of belief. There are beliefs that are opinions, and beliefs that are convictions. Someone who is deeply religious has a conviction, which is not usually open to doubt or change. This is stronger than an opinion, because in religion we are taught not to doubt but to accept without question the teachings of whichever religion we follow. Don't make your beliefs so rigid that you can't change them. Make them opinions rather than convictions so that you *can* change them. Be flexible rather than unyielding in what you choose to believe.

Positive or negative thoughts can and will dictate our reality, and self-limiting beliefs can come true, whether based on fact or fiction. We must challenge all negative beliefs about pregnancy, since they are not based on facts at all and definitely not based on facts that are relevant to us. Even if you have had several miscarriages, it does not mean you will have another any more than carrying a handicapped child means you will carry another. Annabel Heseltine had three failed pregnancies before having twins using IVF. Then she conceived naturally and had a third baby the following year, followed by a fourth. Yasmin Le Bon had several miscarriages before she went on to have three daughters. Heather Mills had two ectopic pregnancies and was told that even if she conceived, she could not carry a baby due to the damage she sustained when her pelvis was crushed in an accident, but she went on to carry her daughter to full term. Actress Patricia Hodge conceived naturally and completely unexpectedly at forty-two and again at forty-five, after suffering with unexplained infertility for over thirteen years. And there are many more examples like these:

Misconceptions

- Annie Leibovitz was in her fifties when she had her baby through IVF.
- Al Pacino and Beverly D'Angelo had twin boys when she was forty-nine and he was in his early sixties, via IVF.
- Cheryl Tiegs had twins at age fifty-two.
- Helen Fielding had her first child at forty-five and her second child at age forty-eight.
- Arlene Phillips had a second daughter naturally at age forty-eight.
- Geena Davis had her first baby at forty-six and twins at forty-eight, through IVF.
- Kelly Preston had a baby boy at age forty-eight.
- Iman had a daughter with David Bowie at age forty-seven.
- Holly Hunter had twins at age forty-seven.
- Diana Ross and Susan Sarandon both had babies at age forty-six.
- Cherie Blair had Leo at age forty-five.
- Jane Seymour and Marcia Cross had twins at age forty-four.
- Meera Syal had a baby naturally at age forty-four.
- Carla Bruni had a baby at age forty-four.
- Sharon Davies had her third child at age forty-four.
- Caroline Quentin gave birth at age forty-three.
- Mariella Frostrup had her children at ages forty-one and forty-two.
- Halle Berry had her first child at forty-one.

- Mariah Carey had twins at forty-one.
- Anna Walker had twins in her forties.
- Bob Champion had testicular cancer, while Lance Armstrong had both testicular and brain cancer. They were each told that they would not be able to father children, and both have since gone on to do so.

Of course there are hundreds of examples of everyday people getting pregnant having been told it was impossible due to their age or health. The number of women in their forties having babies has tripled in the last few years. Although we are led to believe that older mothers are a new phenomenon, women have had late babies through the ages. When women in previous generations had a lot of children, they would start in their late teens and continue into their late thirties. If a woman had her first baby at eighteen and went on to have twelve or more children (which was not uncommon some time ago), she would generally have had them about eighteen months apart, so women having babies in their late thirties and early forties is nothing new. The famous poet Elizabeth Browning Barrett gave birth to her son in 1849, when she was forty-three years old, and biologically she would have been much older than a forty-three-year-old today, and she suffered with very poor health all her life.

With every belief you have about your fertility, it is important to ask yourself, 'Where did that belief come from? What authority did the person who passed that belief to me have? Where did they get it from, and is it relevant to me? Is it based on anything that is real and tangible?' You may surprise yourself with some of your answers.

Beliefs related to fertility are changing all the time. Young women may have more energy to raise a child, but older women have more patience and wisdom and

Misconceptions

tend not to focus on missing out on a social life. Older women have traditionally raised young children when young mothers depended on older female relations to help, as they had to work.

Beliefs affect everything. The most important are identity beliefs. A very strong force in humans is the need to remain consistent with how we define ourselves, and those beliefs can be empowering or limiting depending on how we formulate them.

We know that unexplained infertility can occur in very young women, and it is not related to age at all. Beliefs actually create biology. There is nothing in the world more powerful than thought. No drug exists that is stronger than the mind. Beliefs are physical and real, but unfortunately, most people are completely unaware of the power of the mind. Unless you take charge of your beliefs, you will act and react to beliefs fed to you by others, which may have no relevance to you.

Since I want you to use the power of your mind to improve your fertility and your chances of having a baby, I am going to spend some of this Step proving to you just how powerful your mind is, so that you can use it to increase your fertility.

Baby Exercises: 2.

By completing this very simple exercise, you will be able to experience how your beliefs cause physical changes to occur within your body.

Stand up. With one arm, pointing your finger out in front of you, begin to move your arm as far out and behind you as you can. If it's your right arm move it out to the right, if it's your left move it out to the left. When you have moved your arm as far behind you as you can, look behind you to notice where it is.

Now, return to the starting position. Close your eyes for a moment, and just imagine your arm moving 25 per cent farther. Really see this in your mind for a moment, and tell yourself that when you repeat the exercise your arm *will* move 25 per cent farther. Then open your eyes, repeat the procedure, and notice just how much farther your arm will move.

You are already beginning to see the power of beliefs on the body. As you saw, believed, and thought about your arm moving farther, it did. Repeat the exercise with the other arm to prove to yourself how easy it is to influence your body using your belief system.

Athletes have been using this technique for years, seeing themselves: lifting a heavier weight, performing a longer jump, believing they will do it, can do it, and then doing exactly that. Many tests have proven that in athletics, the ability to visualise is as important as physical training. When athletes visualise, they cause all their muscles to perform at a level to meet the visualisation. It is now becoming accepted that athletes who use powers of visualisation, as well as training, will always achieve more.

I once made a television documentary with some of my clients who are Olympic athletes. They were talking about how many athletes at the last Olympic Games used the power of thought, belief, and visualisation to succeed, and how it gave them an advantage over those who didn't, often helping them break a world record.

You may have heard stories of people who are slightly built or unfit, lifting a heavy object like a car, tree, or refrigerator off their child who is trapped underneath, and then wondering how they managed it. In fact, they momentarily *saw* themselves performing the feat and then performed it, because in their mind, in that moment, they believed they could and would do it. One of the rules of the mind is 'Imagination is more powerful than logic.' Reason can be overruled by imagination, and you can use this to your advantage as you believe in your ability to improve your fertility...and then make it a reality. People who see themselves as being ill, who believe they *are* ill, can and do manifest all the symptoms of illness, whereas people who refuse to see themselves as ill or who won't believe they are unwell frequently defy medical opinions. People who are ill and see themselves recovering, and use their imagination to see cells becoming healthy, dwelling on wellness instead of illness, tend to recover much more rapidly and more frequently than those who use the same powers of imagination and belief to focus on what is wrong with them.

A phantom pregnancy is an obvious example of thoughts and beliefs in the mind creating physical changes in the body. During a phantom pregnancy, breasts can produce milk, the stomach will swell and, should the phantom pregnancy continue to full term, labour can begin, although only blood is passed. Adoptive mothers are able to lactate and breast feed an adopted baby by visualising milk flowing to their breasts, and by wearing formula milk in a pouch with a tube running to their nipple, so as the baby sucks the milk, it sends a powerful message to the brain to make more for the feeding baby. One of my clients, who adopted a three-week-old baby from South America, immediately felt such love for the baby that she noticed when she was taking a bath the following week, milk began to pour from her breasts, and she had not even been on the lactating programme.

Another fascinating example of the power of belief on the body is that of people with multiple personality disorders, where one personality may have allergies, need glasses, or have arthritis, while another personality within the same person, is completely free of these needs and afflictions. Some female multiple personalities have even switched on and off their periods depending on which personality they are experiencing. These studies show us that cells are intelligent and make choices about how to behave below the level of our awareness.

Every cell in your body has its own micro brain, and unlike your brain, which has learnt to doubt, and may doubt your ability when you say, 'I am expecting a baby' or 'I am becoming a mother,' cells have no ability to doubt what we tell them. If you constantly tell yourself you are very fertile and expecting to have a baby, you are more likely to overcome unexplained infertility, because your body, and in particular, your reproductive system, will believe you and will act accordingly. Your cells and your body respond to what you believe, and beliefs change all the time, yet so many people condition themselves by believing things that are outdated and inappropriate. It used to be believed that having our teeth, appendix, and tonsils removed as a matter of routine was beneficial, but now that belief has changed, and we have been made aware it can be harmful to remove organs for no reason. When false teeth first originated, they were a status symbol, and some young, wealthy people had all their teeth removed and replaced with false ones because of this belief. In the early twentieth century, it was fashionable for young, wealthy brides to be given a full set of false teeth as a wedding present from their fathers-in-law.[10]

---

10 www.bda-dentistry.org.uk

Misconceptions

So many beliefs based on medical opinions change, because new discoveries and facts come to light. This is certainly true with fertility. In 1999, a baby who was one of triplets developed perfectly outside his mother's womb while his siblings grew in the womb. Despite being given a one in sixty million chance of survival, baby Ronan, who began life as an ectopic pregnancy, grew in his mother's abdominal cavity, and was delivered at thirty-two weeks, weighing two pounds, one ounce, and is now a healthy boy, along with his two triplet siblings.

An Italian woman made history by becoming pregnant a second time when she was already several months pregnant. When Mandy Allwood was carrying eight babies in 1996, the medical profession stated it was not possible for a woman to carry eight babies to a stage where they could safely be born, because as the babies grew larger, her womb would ultimately expel them all. They warned Mandy that unless she terminated some of her babies she would lose all of them, and that is sadly exactly what happened. Yet in 1998, Nkem Chukwu, from Texas, gave birth to eight babies, seven of which survived and are perfectly healthy. In 2009, Nadya Suleman birthed eight babies. So in just two years, what was accepted as a medical fact (that the womb could not carry eight babies) is no longer true, that's how quickly medical opinions can change.

You can improve your fertility by changing your beliefs, and you can improve your chances of having a baby by removing preconditioned beliefs that do not apply to you.

In undeveloped countries, married couples don't try to prevent conception, and they have little or no negativity attached to having a baby. In the Western world, we have a different awareness about pregnancy, but you can use this awareness to your advantage by choosing not to believe that having a baby is a journey loaded with problems and complications. Instead choose to believe that you can positively influence your pregnancy, your baby, and its birth. During the next few days and weeks, become aware of any self-limiting beliefs you hold regarding motherhood, and remember they may exist only in your imagination since you can usually find examples to counteract these beliefs. You can replace any negative beliefs about having a baby with positive beliefs. The mind can only hold one thought at a time, so you must banish negative beliefs and replace them with positive ones. You can choose what to believe. Your relatives' beliefs don't have to be relevant for you. What about your friends' beliefs? Do they match your own? Do you go along with what they say just because they said it?

Close your eyes, and just allow yourself to hear all the things you have heard from your family, your friends, and the media, about having a baby. Have you heard that birth is agony, that you never get your figure back, that you will forget what it was like to have a good night's sleep, let alone a sex life? Have you heard that you will look haggard and worn out, that your husband will be jealous of the baby, that you won't be able to give him lots of attention, and that he will leave you for some nubile young thing? Babies scream for hours, and there is nothing you can do about it. Have you heard that your life won't be your own again for years, if ever, and you will be permanently broke because babies cost an extortionate sum to raise.

You do not have to believe any of these things if you don't want to. Birth can be a wonderful experience. Your baby's birth day can be the most wonderful day of your life. It certainly was for me. I had an easy birth and an easy baby who didn't cry much at all. She was a dream, and I was very happy. In the hospital, my friends, some of whom where pregnant with their first babies, came to visit and immediately began asking me questions such as, 'So, how was it? Are you exhausted? Do you have post-natal depression? Does she cry all the time? Were you in agony? Did you get any sleep at all?' In fact, I was never exhausted. I had post-natal euphoria, and I was on such a high when I had my baby because I conditioned and programmed myself to feel that way. Maybe I was incredibly lucky, but I planned it to be that way by expecting to feel euphoric and visualising myself feeling wonderful and elated by my daughter's birth. I talked to my baby in the womb all the time and told her to sleep at night. I told myself I would gain a healthy weight and lose it easily afterwards. My sister had already told me that new-borns are easy to raise because they sleep so much, and my mother told me it was wonderful having a new baby to care for. Maybe I sound sickeningly glib, but all the mothers I work with tell me that expecting to feel euphoric and seeing themselves as a natural mother instinctively caring for their baby works for them. I have only ever had one patient who experienced post-natal depression, and after working with her, it disappeared completely.

To this day I dislike press articles talking about the difficulties in store for new mothers, emphasising that it takes hours to get ready in the morning, that it's often impossible to get out of the house or even get dressed, let alone take a shower, and that a baby causes major stress. That may be the case if you have two or three young children, but one small baby does not disrupt a house, and in fact brings such joy. I think that articles exaggerating the stress and woes of motherhood are very damaging and irresponsible. They are telling women that one of the most magical times in your life, when you have a wonderful new-born baby, is non-stop stress. If it were really that bad, we wouldn't do it a second or third time. In the age of washing machines, dryers, freezers, instant heating, baby clothes that never need ironing, stores that deliver anything and everything, and healthy food that's easy to prepare, women today have it much easier than their predecessors. Sleep deprivation can be a problem, but if you only have one child, you can sleep whenever he or she sleeps, and wear clothes you don't need to iron. The effect of all this moaning and scaremongering in the press is that it can subconsciously cause you to link pain rather than pleasure to having a baby. As I have mentioned before, your brain's job is to prevent you from experiencing anything you link pain to.

Baby Exercises: 3.

Using your notebook, write a list of attitudes and beliefs about having a baby you have taken on board from people who could have influenced you, and which you are now ready to change. Underneath each one, write down something new, positive, and appropriate for you.

For example:
'My mother always told me that having a baby meant losing your figure forever, and being fat with droopy breasts.'

Underneath you might write:
'Jerry Hall, Trudi Styler, Heidi Klum, and Sadie Frost have all given birth four times and retained stunning figures. Jane Seymour has four children, including twins she had at forty-five. Diana Ross has five children; she had the last two in her mid-forties. Kate Winslet was thinner than she had ever been a year after having her second child.'

These examples are of the rich and famous, but many ordinary women do exactly the same. The only reason I refer to famous women is so that you can use them as examples that will help you to change your thinking.

Here are some more examples:
'My grandmother believed that birth was terrifying and agonising, and that you could die giving birth.'

Change to:
'I will have a wonderful birth because I can choose what type of birth I want, and I can benefit from all the advances in medicine and obstetrics available to me.'

Death in childbirth is now rare and pain management is so far advanced from when our grandmothers gave birth.

Or:

'What if I am a terrible mother and my baby doesn't like me, or I don't like it?'

Change to:

'My baby will be a part of me, and I will love it. There are so many books, CDs, and courses available to help me be a good parent.'

Or:

'I don't want to be fat for nine months and have no control of my body.'

Change to:

'I will be pregnant, not fat, and pregnancy can look beautiful. My body will not be out of control. Pregnancy is not an illness, it's a natural state.

Next, decide what you are going to believe in relation to having your baby, and write out these new beliefs. Accept them as your beliefs from now on. Remember, you can influence and improve your chances of having a baby depending on what you choose to believe, what you choose to hold in your mind as true or not true, and what you choose to see as relevant or irrelevant to you.

In Step one you discovered and confronted your own thoughts about birth and pregnancy. In Step two, you've learned to discover and confront the beliefs about having a child, which have been passed on to you by the media and by other people. So that you were able to analyse where these beliefs came from, how you got them, and why you believed them. Some of these may be the same or very similar, but even if you find yourself repeating things, keep going, because the mind learns by repetition, and it is important to release every negative thought and belief before you move on to Step three.

You have also proved to yourself, again, with the physical exercises, the power your beliefs have over your body, which will incentivise you to change beliefs that are harmful to you.

"Words form the thread on which we string our experiences."

Aldous Huxley.

STEP THREE:

Baby Talk

The way we talk about babies, pregnancy, and birth, and the language we use, sends a message to our brain telling it what we really feel about being pregnant, giving birth, and raising children. Your mind absolutely influences your body, but it is *your* mind, and *you* have the power to direct it and influence it in the most positive way. The quickest way to do this is to stop using negative words.

If you accept the real and physical effects of your words and your language on your mind and body, then you will accept that by replacing negative words with positive ones, your body will respond differently. Language and the words you use associated with having a baby, have a very powerful effect on the body and mind because words have an emotional content, and what we associate with the words we use, influences how we feel about things. Experiments have been done showing that if we take on someone else's emotional vocabulary, we also take on that person's emotional state. It is not a coincidence that calm mothers tend to have calm babies, and stressed, anxious mothers more frequently have babies who pick up the stress and are also anxious. Calm mothers tend to use calm phrases like, 'It's fine, don't worry, it's not important,' whereas anxious mothers use phrases like, 'It's driving me mad, I'm going crazy, this is stressing me out.' There are many negative words used about pregnancy, words such as fat, exhausted, weepy, emotional, drained, shattered, worn out, and hormonal. Lactating women sometimes say they feel like a cow, like a milk bar, but other women think it is fabulous to have full round breasts and love the experience of feeding their baby. (Natasha Hamilton from Atomic Kitten said it was worth being pregnant for the breasts alone.) Some women imagine that nursing a baby is horrible, whereas others believe it is the most wonderful and beautiful thing, and will breast feed for as long as possible to savour the experience. Every time you feed your baby, you make oxytocin-the 'feel good' hormone. Breast-feeding can hurt initially, but nipple shields are amazingly helpful. For me they made breast-feeding easy and stopped all soreness completely.

When it comes to the birth, using words and phrases like agony, unbearable, unendurable pain, ripped in half, trying to push out a melon, don't help anyone. Eliminate words like tired, exhausted, worn out, shattered, desperate, hormonal, and post-natal depression, because the words you use to describe how you feel can *become* how you feel. Pregnancy can be tiring, but it's also natural, and your body will recover easily with rest.

Your brain uses the words you are speaking to interpret how you are feeling. If you are going through IVF, avoid words and phrases like invasive procedures, low chance of success, painful procedures, humiliating, demeaning, overwhelming, hormonal nightmare, painful injections, or cripplingly expensive. Don't expect it not to work or believe it has only a low or slight chance of working. You can make it more effective by being positive about the whole procedure. Our mind loves and responds to words that are descriptive. Now that you know this, only use descriptive words that are positive. Since words are the structure of our reality, it follows that if we change our words, we can change our reality. Certainly making changes to the language we use changes how we feel very quickly, and that's why it's so important to pay attention to the words and language we use connected to having a baby. Your body will react to your language, so if you are going through IVF whilst telling yourself you are old, your eggs are sparse, old, or of poor quality, you are not helping yourself. However, making very simple changes to your language and saying, 'I am producing plenty of healthy, strong premium grade-A eggs' will have a different effect on your body. After all, you only need one superior egg and one superior sperm to make a baby.

If your language and thoughts are all along the lines of 'I can't get pregnant' or 'I can't carry a baby to full term' or 'All the women in our family suffered a dreadful, long labour or got really fat when they were pregnant and never lost the weight again,' you are passing on that information to your body. Your body is not able to disagree with you, and accepts everything you say and think as a fact, so you have nothing to lose and everything to gain by telling yourself only positive things. Tell yourself you are super fertile with strong eggs and healthy hormones, that you are able to sail through pregnancy and are blooming with health, and you will have a positive birth experience. Even if this has not been your experience in the past, your body changes constantly, and you can influence the changes in a positive way by changing your language, thoughts, and beliefs.

In the area of language, the word *loss* is a painful one. All human pain is linked to loss, so if you equate being pregnant with losing your figure, losing your independence, and losing your freedom, or if you see being a mother as losing your lifestyle, your tidy, neat home, or intimate moments with your husband, that is what will manifest. Even if you jokingly say things like, 'It will never be the same again, I won't be able to see my feet for nine months. I will never get into my jeans or be a size ten again,' or worry that you may lose your position at work during maternity leave, or that you will be unable to leave your baby to return to work, or ever find the right childcare again, you will accelerate your mind into linking more pain than pleasure to being a mother.

Gain is a positive word, where *loss* is negative, so change your vocabulary, focus on gaining a baby and gaining so much love, pleasure, and happiness in making a family, creating a new life, and loving the miracle of watching and feeling your baby grow inside you. Think about that momentous event when you give birth and meet this perfect person that you made.

Someone once told me if they could have their life to live over that '*Instead of wishing away nine months of pregnancy, I'd have cherished every moment and realised that the wonderment growing inside me was the only chance in life to assist God in a miracle.*'

If you are undergoing IVF, accept you are going through a process that can be challenging, but is worth it to have a baby. Do not focus on the time, the procedures, or the statistics. Instead focus on the fact that when your eggs are collected, fertilised, and then put back in you, you are pregnant, and you have a huge power to influence your future baby at every stage of IVF, especially during the embryo transfer. Remember, most IVF statistics apply to the embryo transfer. The chances of you ovulating healthy eggs with IVF are higher than 25 per cent. Your chances of those eggs being fertilised with IVF or ICSI are higher than 25 per cent, but it reduces to 25 per cent at implantation. This is when many women become nervous that it won't work, instead of focusing on helping it to work and connecting to the intelligence of the embryo.

It's very important to remember that having good eggs is the key for both natural and IVF conception. We know that women in their sixties can carry babies to full term and deliver healthy babies because several women in their late sixties have done this by using donated eggs. We also know that when women freeze their eggs or embryos and later fertilise those eggs, the age of the eggs or embryos is far more important than the age of her womb and all the risk is carried in the age of the eggs, not in the age of the woman's body as the uterus is nearly ageless. So it's very important to visualise your eggs as young and grade-A perfect. This is absolutely possible, as the age of your ovaries can be several years younger than your actual age.

Sophia Loren and Belinda Carlisle spent almost their entire pregnancies in bed. Sophia Loren did it a second time with her next son and said she did not expect to be applauded for it, as it was worth every moment to have a healthy child. An American woman who was carrying multiple babies had to spend almost five months lying upside down, using gravity to prevent her womb from expelling the babies. She said selective abortion did not exist in her vocabulary, and she would not choose which babies to give up, as nowhere in her Bible told her how to do this. She would have them all because she had been given them all, and she did it, because she willingly lay inverted for five months in order to have her children. In 2011 a British woman Donna Kelly spent ten weeks, 24 hours a day, lying 'upside down' in a hospital bed until she gave birth to a healthy daughter, Amelia. Some women have done amazing things in order to have children…because it's worth it.

Baby Exercises: 4.

Why can't I have a baby? Versus I am young and fertile and expecting a baby.

You will need someone to help you do this. Stand on the ground with your feet a few inches apart and your arms by your side. Now get your helper to push you while you keep your feet firmly planted on the ground and resist the pushing.

Now that you have established your strength, think of the most negative words or beliefs you use about yourself in relation to having a baby. Repeat these words out loud ten times, or just think them silently, ten times. An example might be: 'I am running out of time to conceive' or 'I have left it for too long, and my eggs are no good.'

Now, thinking these thoughts let your helper push you again. You will notice that you lose your balance and step backwards. Amazing, isn't it? As you think those negative thoughts, you lose your balance and become weaker. This is even more proof of the amazing powers of the mind.

This time, think of some positive thoughts about your fertility and your ability to have a baby. Repeat them silently, or out loud, ten times. A good example might be: 'I am super fertile. My reproductive system is excellent. I am expecting a baby.'

Still thinking these thoughts, let your helper push you again, and you will find that you can resist and stay strongly rooted to the ground. Isn't it great to see that as you think positive thoughts you become physically stronger? I mentioned earlier that every thought you have creates a physical reaction in the body, and you have just proved it to yourself.

I always tell my patients that they are expecting a baby, and that they are a mother-to-be, even before they are pregnant, as once you connect with the life force of your baby and talk to it, visualise it, and take action to conceive it, you can think of yourself as a mother-to-be. You can expect a baby in the same way you expect a letter, phone call, or your yearly tax bill. It may not have arrived yet, but you believe and know it is on its way to you.

Where a thought goes, energy goes with it, so changing your thinking and using different language really does change your body. Most people are fascinated by this testing, and since it's a fun thing to do, I recommend you spend some time playing with it.

Repeat all the negative thoughts and beliefs you have, using all the negative words you had been using before you understood the power of language. Then test your strength. Now replace those beliefs with positive constructive beliefs, and test your strength again to see the difference.

You can do this with so many beliefs, not just fertility. You can apply it to beliefs about your confidence, self-esteem, habits, abilities, relationships...anything at all.

You can do the same test with your grip. Push your index finger against your thumb and press really hard while someone tries to prise your fingers apart. Do the same test while thinking negative thoughts and notice how weak your grip becomes and how easy it is for your helper to prise apart your finger and thumb. Now think positive thoughts. Evoke positive statements about your fertility, and notice how much harder (maybe even impossible) it is for your helper to prise apart your grip while you think and speak positive statements.

Remember, these beliefs only exist in your imagination, and you are free to change your thinking and your language as soon as you become aware of how limiting and destructive they are. After all, your thoughts are yours to change, your mind is yours to direct, and your beliefs and language are yours to alter. While the mind does influence the body, it is *your* mind, and you are able to direct it, change it, and use it to influence positive changes in yourself. Changing your language is one of the quickest ways to do this.

Baby Exercises: 5.

I want you to think of all the words and language you use to describe yourself. Write down all the words on a page of your notebook, and then go through them and delete all the words that are not positive. As you delete them, replace each negative word with a new and more appropriate one, or just erase it from your vocabulary.

Examples of negative words might include: infertile, dried up, past it, tired, fat, frazzled, exhausted, emotional, worn out, shattered, depressed, sexless, and barren. Even if you only use the words jokingly, remember our subconscious mind has no sense of humour and takes everything we say literally.

It's important to laugh and to have a sense of humour, and it is okay to make fun of yourself, but not in connection to your fertility. Delete all these words and/or find new words to replace them.

There are 750,000 words in the English language, and most of us only use twelve hundred of them. Most people use the same twelve words to describe all their experiences and feelings. It is especially interesting to me that many people use very descriptive and powerful words to describe events that are ordinary, and use words that are not powerful enough to describe good things that are happening to them.

Sometimes a patient will arrive at my office and say, 'I've had a horrendous morning on the motorway,' or 'The parking around here is a nightmare,' or 'I've been stuck in the supermarket, its hell in there,' or even 'I've had the most torturous time getting here.' Then just for good measure, they will add, 'My back is *killing* me,' or 'I have *starved* myself all week, but I still look as fat as a house.' Without realising it, they are using very powerful, descriptive words to describe events that aren't really that important and need to be forgotten, not elevated, or even remembered in the mind.

Describing pain as *killing* can only intensify it. Saying you are 'ravenous' or 'starved' will cause you to overeat, because your mind will believe you are starving. When these same clients talk about good events in their life or how they are feeling, they use words that are weak or lack description, like, 'It was quite good,' 'I had a nice time,' 'It turned out all right,' or 'I'm fine.' These words are so vague and bland that they fail to have an impact on the mind. If you want to feel better, use words that are really descriptive, and create a picture that is thrilling or exciting and powerful.

Even the words you place in front of other words will have an effect on how you feel. This is especially true with swear words, which are used to intensify a feeling. If you say, 'It was awful,' but add in front of that it was *absolutely* awful, *bloody* awful, *positively* awful or *absolutely bloody* awful, your mind and body will respond that much more strongly. If you say it was 'amazing,' then make it *truly* amazing, *simply* amazing, *absolutely* amazing, you will react more strongly (positively) to the event.

If you are undergoing fertility treatment, don't think of it as agonising, humiliating, or degrading. When you think of giving birth, don't think of it as excruciating, agonising, terrifying, or unbearable. Instead, think of it as challenging, bearable, durable, and only slightly uncomfortable, because these words are minimal in description, and you will cope much better.

Think about the words and language you use in connection to pregnancy and childbirth. Write them out, and then minimise the negative and accentuate the positive.

Examples:

Replace: *I won't be able to endure the pain.*
With: *I will cope beautifully.*
Replace: *I will hate being fat.*
With: *Pregnancy looks very beautiful.*
Replace: *I hate hospitals, even the smell, and I don't want to be in one.*
With: *A delivery room is nothing like an operating theatre.*

Now think of the words you use in front of other words, and use adverbs like *absolutely, definitely, positively, unquestionably*, and so on, in front of your new positive statements. Don't use words with a strong negative emotional content, like, 'I am desperate to get pregnant,' or 'I dread giving birth,' or 'I can't bear to think of an epidural,' or 'I loathe the thought of all those embarrassing, intimate examinations,' because the more descriptive and negative those words are, the more they will elevate, negatively, how you feel about having a baby, despite the fact that you really want one. What our mind sees it believes without question.

The mind has no capacity to reason. It believes whatever it is told. Get into the habit of telling yourself only positive things. Also get into the habit of being very aware of the language, the words you use to describe things, especially when describing yourself, because your mind particularly responds to words and images that are symbolic. The subconscious mind loves descriptive words.

If you say, 'I am fertile' or 'I am super fertile,' your mind first creates a picture of what that means, and then works to make you feel and act in ways that match those pictures. If you say, 'I have crippling back pain' or 'I have excruciating mastitis,' your body works to meet the mind's description. Simply changing that to 'I have mild discomfort in my back' or 'My breasts feel uncomfortable' will eventually bring about completely different sensations. Rather than saying, 'I am really anxious and worried about the birth,' you can say, 'I am concerned about some aspects of it.'

When I hypnotise clients to help them give birth, I remove the words *labour, pain* and *contractions* from the conditioning tape I make for them, and instead talk about *delivery, birth signals, rushes, feelings, sensations, euphoria.* Many of my clients who listen to this tape during the last stages of pregnancy and during delivery say they love it because it contains no negative words and allows them to experience childbirth in a more manageable way.

When I was pregnant, I was amazed that my antenatal clinic wanted to remind me at every visit to be prepared for postnatal depression. They even went so far as to say that all the mothers on the ward would cry in tandem by day four. I would always reply, 'I am going to have postnatal euphoria.' Eventually I stopped going, because they always seemed to talk about the pain of birth, the baby blues, the complications involved in breast feeding, and the exhaustion of being a new mother. They told me that the pain was often unbearable, and new mothers were exhausted and weepy during the first few weeks. I had a very easy pregnancy and birth, and I did have postnatal euphoria. I felt incredibly well after my baby's birth, so I left the hospital after day two, just to make sure I was not around all the weeping. I took my daughter out for a walk when she was three days old, and several people told me my baby and I should be at home in bed, as if we were both ill. I had a very easy pregnancy and birth because I conditioned myself to believe different things. I used positive language and positive thoughts. I also had further motivation to do this, as I went on live television three weeks after my baby's birth to demonstrate hypnosis for childbirth on a woman who was phobic about hospitals, and I took my baby with me. I was regarded as something of an exception because I returned to my normal weight very quickly, and I felt fantastic. I still believe that a lot of the things we hear about pregnancy, such as the weight that takes a year to disappear, the tiredness, the depression, promotes negative conditioning that many women react to automatically because of the way the mind works. Of course some women do experience postnatal depression, but you can decide that this will not apply to you. You may need to persist with changing your language and vocabulary if you have been using powerful, negative words relating to conception and pregnancy for some time. The mind learns by repetition, so get into the habit of repeating positive words and phrases about having your baby.

To feel more in control of your fertility, you must change your attitudes, your assumptions, your awareness, and your language about having a baby. There is so much you can do to take control of your baby's conception and birth that there is no need to feel helpless about it. It is very normal for humans to fear change at some level, just in case it's for the worst, but you can learn to influence the direction of change in your life and make it change for the better, especially when these changes relate to your body and lifestyle that pregnancy and motherhood bring. Once you do this, your mind and body will welcome the changes rather than fear them. You will begin to feel so much more positive when you know that you are influencing the direction of change in your life and realise that you can positively influence every change that having a baby will bring to you.

I could write an entire book on my experiences with clients who changed their thoughts and beliefs and created wonderful changes within themselves, but I will describe just a few for you. Mrs Drew was a delightful American woman who came to see me while she was in England for a few weeks. She had been trying to get pregnant for thirteen years and had done almost everything, including many attempts at IVF. Eventually she gave up and was able to arrange privately to adopt a baby from a young single mother who was pregnant. Mrs Drew was in London with her husband a month before the baby was due and she came to see me for hypnosis to deal with some personal issues before taking charge of her new baby. Obviously she was very excited and would arrive at my office with all kinds of baby clothes and toys, which she had bought on the way, and she would show me her purchases while we talked about her impending motherhood. Her joy and delight were contagious. However, while in London she received a phone call telling her that the baby had been born a month early. The mother could not bear to part with her, so the adoption would not be going ahead. Mrs Drew was devastated, and she stayed on in England for a few extra weeks, unable to face returning to her home where the baby's room was decorated and filled with toys waiting for her arrival. I did a lot of work with her until she felt able to return to America, determined to keep going and eventually adopt another baby.

Five weeks after her return, she called me to say that she was pregnant. In fact, she had been pregnant whilst in England, but had no idea. It seemed like the most wonderful miracle. While she was focusing on becoming a mother, she got pregnant, and at last had her baby. While she was buying things for her baby and talking about the baby she was expecting, her body made a baby in response to her expectations.

Many women who want children focus on why they can't get pregnant. They say things like, 'Why can't I have a baby? What's wrong with me? Why is my body letting me down? It's so unfair!' They hope, wish, and pray for motherhood.

Mrs Drew, unaware of what she was doing, actually focused on being a mother. She talked about her baby, shopped for her baby, decorated the baby's room, and completely accepted herself as a mother. She saw herself as a mother rather than wishing, hoping, and longing to become one. She showed anyone who expressed an interest all the things she was buying for *her* baby.

Couples who have adopted often go on to have children naturally after the adoption is completed and sometimes even when the adoption process is still underway. It has been said it is because they become relaxed about it when they know they will have their baby through adoption. I believe it is because, unquestionably, they see themselves and accept themselves as parents. Like Mrs Drew, they prepare themselves and their homes for a child's arrival...not wishing it would arrive, but absolutely *knowing* it is on its way.

You want to have a baby, so instead of wishing, hoping, longing for, or dreaming of it, see it as if you already have it. Believe it is happening for you now, as the mind only works in the present tense. *Know* that it will happen instead of *hoping* it will happen. When you wish for something, you send a message to the brain that says, 'I want this, but I don't believe I can ever have it.' When you say, 'I will try,' your brain immediately accepts the word 'try' as so insignificant that it does not matter if you get the results or not, and when you say *I will* instead of *I'll try*, you get a very different and positive response.

Saying 'I hope it works' allows your mind to believe that you doubt it will work. Saying 'I dream about being pregnant' is interpreted by the mind as dreaming about something, because you have already accepted that it is not attainable.

Some years ago I was asked to work with a little boy who had eczema. His parents were very keen that he might find a cure for it, while his grandmother, who lived with the family, would comment frequently that they should all stop fussing since it would go away when he started school. I could not give them an appointment until after he had begun his first term at school, as I was out of the country. Interestingly, as soon as he began school, the eczema started to diminish, and by the time he arrived for his appointment it had already improved by 75 per cent because he had accepted his grandmother's words, and his mind had acted upon them without even needing to understand them.

Occasionally clients book appointments to help them stop smoking or nail biting, and then they arrive for the appointment having already stopped, or considerably reduced the habit…because they expected to, and in a sense saw it happening.

I have my own personal experience of the power of thought, as I was told I could not get pregnant, but I did. I was told that my baby could be born with some health issues, so I used hypnosis throughout my pregnancy. I had the easiest pregnancy, an easy birth, and a baby who was perfectly healthy and so content, she hardly ever cried.

In Step three of *Trying to get Pregnant (and Succeeding),* you have learnt the power of language and the real and physical effects of your words on your mind and body. You are almost a third of the way through the programme and are much more in control of your fertility already.

"If you do what you have always done, you get what you have always got."

Mark Twain.

STEP FOUR:

Baby Rules

Understanding the rules of how your mind works will help you to positively influence your mind, rather than being influenced by thoughts, beliefs, and behaviours that you do not want.

Imagine that you purchased a top-of-the-range computer or washing machine and it came without instructions. How would you use it? You might find that you could not use it at all, or you might muddle through, but you would never get the best out of your machine. You could never use it to its full capacity, and you would not get the excellent results that it was capable of giving to you. We come into this world with the most amazing computer-like brain that is capable of doing so much, but there are no instructions given that tell us how to get the best from ourselves, and no manual that shows us how to programme ourselves for success. So we muddle through, when we are capable of so much more. You can find instructions on how to take charge of your body, weight, and shape, but very little on how to run your mind. This is changing slowly, however, and there are some books and courses available now that will point you in the right direction. Some of them are excellent, and I look forward to the day when this information is taught in schools.

Here is a list of the rules of the mind as they apply to fertility. By reading them you will have a greater understanding of yourself. Some of them may seem a little repetitive and cover information that you have already come across in the first three steps, but our mind learns by repetition, so see that as a good thing.

1: Every thought or idea causes a physical reaction.

Thoughts have consequences and create changes in the body. Thoughts create chemical reactions in the body. Ideas that have a strong emotional content always reach the subconscious mind, because it is the *feeling* mind. Once accepted, these ideas create the same reactions in the body again and again. To change negative reactions in the body, it is important to change the ideas responsible for the reaction, both consciously and subconsciously. So if you have strong negative emotions linked to pregnancy and birth, they will move into your subconscious mind and have a very real effect on you. By changing your thoughts so that you have strong, positive emotions linked to pregnancy and birth, you can ensure that the effect your thoughts and emotions have on your body is positive and beneficial.

2: What is expected tends to be realised.

The brain and nervous system respond to mental images, regardless of whether the image is real or imagined. The mental image formed becomes a blueprint, and the subconscious mind uses every means at its disposal to act according to the blueprint. Worrying about not conceiving, or miscarrying, is a form of programming a picture of what we *don't* want (the blueprint), but the subconscious mind acts to fulfil the picture it is seeing. That's why it is so important not to create or hold on to pictures in your mind about what could go wrong in a pregnancy or birth, but decide instead to hold positive images of everything working out perfectly. Our physical health can be absolutely linked to our mental expectancy, so if you expect to have a difficult pregnancy, or if you say, 'I'm bound to gain masses of weight that I can't lose afterwards,' or 'It will be just my luck to have morning sickness all day and a long tiring birth,' then you probably will. Instead of expecting a pregnancy that resembles an illness, remove every despondent and negative attitude about pregnancy and birth, and expect to have a wonderful experience. Expect to maintain and prolong your fertility. If you expect to conceive, carry, and deliver a robustly healthy baby, and expect to take to motherhood with ease, these expectations are more likely to be realised.

3: Imagination is more powerful than knowledge when dealing with your own mind, or the minds of other people.

Reason is easily overruled by imagination. Violence would be unheard of if logic were able to override the emotional reaction. We can all stand on a piece of wood on the floor, but if that piece of wood became a plank placed high up between two buildings, the image of yourself falling would become more powerful than the knowledge that you can stand there if you have to. Any idea accompanied by a strong emotion, such as anger, fear, panic, or jealousy, is more powerful than any logical information meant to counteract it. Your imagination and your ability to see yourself as fertile, to believe you can have a baby, is more powerful than any medical data that says it can't be done. Since science now says it *can* be done, and since there is well-documented proof and examples of women having healthy babies later in life against medical expectations, we really have no reason to fear infertility and childlessness.

4: Each suggestion acted upon lowers opposition to successive suggestions.

Once a suggestion has been accepted by the subconscious mind, it becomes easier for additional suggestions to be accepted and acted upon. So if we assume that this book has already caused you to accept some new suggestions, you can take faith in the knowledge that this alone is making it easier for you, for your mind, to accept further beneficial information about you and your fertility.

5: An emotionally induced symptom will cause organic change if maintained for long enough.

Many doctors have acknowledged that more than 75 per cent of human ailments are functional rather than organic, meaning that the function of an organ or other body part has been disturbed by the nervous system's reaction to negative ideas held in the subconscious mind. We cannot separate the mind from the body, so if you dread the IVF procedure or the idea of birth and hospitals or if you are searching for signs of miscarriage while pregnant, or looking for signs of early menopause while wanting to conceive, then in time negative organic changes must occur. Many women spend the early part of their pregnancy preoccupied with miscarrying and won't buy any baby things in case they 'tempt fate' and miscarry, but in thinking this way they are sending a negative expectation to their mind and body. If you welcome and enjoy every stage of conception, pregnancy, and birth, and expect to produce a thriving healthy baby, then positive organic changes are much more likely to occur.

6: When dealing with the subconscious mind and its functions, the greater the conscious effort, the less the subconscious response.

Willpower is not the right tool to use when implementing change. Haven't we all tried really hard to remember something, yet were unable to do it, and then found that, as we stopped trying, the information we were looking for sprang to mind? This is because the more conscious effort you make, the less the subconscious responds. Trying to go to sleep doesn't work for an insomniac and trying to relax is ineffective for anxious people.

When you are making physical changes by using exercise, it's true that the more effort you put in, the more results you will get back, but when you are making mental changes, when you are changing your thoughts, beliefs, and expectations, the opposite applies. You don't need to try you just need to let your subconscious absorb these new ideas. Let your mind accept them by being open to them. When making mental changes, effort is not truly necessary. What is necessary is the ability to get an image of how you plan to be (pregnant, or relaxing with your perfect new born) and to hold that image in your mind. Relax into the image, and use language that matches it. Keep re-running the image so you are rehearsing it to such an extent that your brain thinks, 'I have been here before. I know how to do this; it is easy.' As you take on new beliefs about your fertility, you will replace all the old negative ones, but you must do it fully and programme your subconscious mind specifically. So, form good images about pregnancy, birth, and raising a baby, in your subconscious mind, which is the feeling mind, and is able to remove, alter, or amend older negative ideas and beliefs.

7: Once an idea has been accepted by the subconscious mind, it remains there until it is replaced by another idea.

(The companion rule to this is)

8: The longer the idea remains the more opposition there is to replacing it with a new idea.

Once an idea has been accepted, it tends to remain. The longer it is held, the more it tends to become a fixed way of thinking. This is how habits of action are formed, both good and bad. First is the habit of thought and then the habit of action. We have habits of thinking as well as habits of action, but the thought always comes first. Therefore, if we want to change our actions, we must begin by changing our thoughts. The poet, John Dryden, said, "*We first make our habits, and then our habits make us.*"

We have many thought habits that are incorrect, but are still fixed in the mind. Every time you used birth control, you were sending a message to your mind loud and clear: *I don't want a baby*. This is not necessarily true now. It was only true at that particular time in your life, but the idea is still there, and it becomes a fixed habit of thought. The mind might experience opposition when trying to replace it with a correct idea. These are fixed ideas, not fleeting thoughts, but no matter how fixed the ideas are or how long they have been held, they can be changed. All beliefs, even very strong beliefs, can be changed if you introduce doubt, because the minute you begin to question something, you no longer really believe it. If you ask someone if her partner is faithful, she will have a belief or a conviction, but if you suggest to her that you know otherwise, that you have information that her partner is seeing someone else, you might place doubt in her mind. It very much depends on the person's belief system. Now look at all your beliefs about fertility and how you believe you will cope with being pregnant, giving birth, and raising children. Are they negative beliefs or very positive ones? You will find all the information you need, in this book, to allow you to introduce doubt into any unhelpful or negative belief, conviction, or opinion about making babies.

9: The mind cannot hold conflicting beliefs.

The mind cannot hold conflicting thoughts, either. We can't be honest and dishonest at the same time, or happy and sad simultaneously. If you hold conflicting beliefs, it sends the mind into a spin and blocks it from moving you towards what it is that you really want.

Making jokes about the supposed horrors of pregnancy and birth, and exaggerating what we perceive giving birth does to us while longing to have a baby are examples of conflicting beliefs. You cannot plan to have a wonderful pregnancy and then engage in joking about the awfulness of it, because the beliefs are contradictory. They confuse the mind, which has to take everything you say as the literal truth. I mentioned earlier that we are controlled by what we link pain and pleasure to. People who are successful in any area, such as relationships, health, or career, have very clear definitions. For example, if you long to have a baby but fear a miscarriage or becoming vulnerable while pregnant, or one day being rejected by your child, then you are linking pleasure and pain to the same thing, and your mind can't move towards pleasure and away from pain, because they are linked to the same event...in this instance, having a baby. If you want to be a mother but link pain to having to give up your career or not having your weekends free, then you have mixed associations, which you must change. Pain is always the more dominant emotion and your mind will do more to avoid pain than it will to get pleasure because avoiding pain is how we survive on the planet.

Bulimics are an interesting example of mixed associations, because they link both pain and pleasure to food. They hate being full and yet love being full. They love food, and they detest even the smell of it. They love the feeling of having an empty stomach, and they loathe it. They usually think of food all day, yet want to be indifferent to food, often reading cookery books, yet not wanting to eat. Changing your associations makes life so much easier, and humans are the only creatures lucky enough to be able to choose what to associate pain or pleasure to. It has been said that this ability is a major advantage and equal disadvantage to being human. I can choose to love eating meat or to link pain to it and thus become a vegetarian, but I would find it hard if I linked pleasure to meat whilst deciding to give it up. If I hate exercising and link pain to it but feel I have to do it, it will always be a chore, but if I decide I *want* to exercise, and that I will enjoy it, it becomes more of a pleasure.

Whatever changes you make as a result of reading this book, make sure you link pleasure to them. If you give up caffeine and alcohol to improve your chances of conception, but resent doing it, your mind will link pain to healthy eating. You might always feel deprived instead of knowing that you have made some fertility-enhancing choices and are feeling great and proud about them.

When you make these changes, don't say 'I *must*,' 'I *have* to,' or 'I have *got* to.' Instead, say, 'I *want* to' or 'I have *chosen* to.' It is such a simple change, and yet it makes such a big difference.

When I was first working on this book, I had some resistance to spending my weekends writing. Friends would invite me over, and I would say, 'I can't, I have to write my book,' yet when I began to say, 'I *want* to write this weekend' or 'I *have chosen to* spend this weekend writing,' I felt entirely different, and I noticed I was enjoying the process.

I hypnotise a lot of students around examination time, and I always tell them that they have *chosen* to study, and that for this particular month they *want* to revise, that it is compelling, that they actually enjoy the process, and that it makes them feel so good to do the work. They almost always send in friends who say, 'You hypnotised my friend to study, and it's amazing, he's actually enjoying it! Can you do the same for me, please?'

If you make a point of linking massive pleasure to the changes you are implementing by filling up your mind with good thoughts, words, and pictures, you will move towards the changes more easily. In the same way, you can link pleasure to every stage of having a baby. Be thrilled and excited about being at home with a new-born. See yourself as a natural, instinctive mother. When we hold small babies, we pat them and rock them instinctively, so see yourself as adapting to motherhood really easily and loving the process. You are able to choose how you feel so don't link pain or fear to having a baby, or you will delay and even block the process. You cannot plan to have a baby while dreading or holding on to fears about what having a baby involves.

Baby Exercises: 6.

Imagine your brain is like a computer screen divided into two columns, headed 'pleasure' and 'pain.' Under the heading of 'pain' are negative pictures and words about pregnancy and babies while under the heading of 'pleasure' are positive images and words about pregnancy and babies.

Now imagine making the 'pleasure' column bigger, brighter, and more joyful, using good words and images link huge, enormous amounts of pleasure to being radiantly pregnant, to having a wonderful birth, and to being a good mother. Use positive pictures and words to create beautiful images of you looking and feeling good at every stage of your pregnancy, the birth, and your parenting.

Now imagine yourself looking at the 'pain' section, seeing all the pain you unconsciously linked to being pregnant, giving birth, or being alone with a baby. Then erase this section completely, just as you would on your computer screen. Delete it all completely.

Your mind is programmed to move you towards pleasure and away from pain, and it will always do much more to avoid pain than it will to seek pleasure. This is why so many people won't risk talking to a stranger they are attracted to, or ask someone for help. The pain of possible rejection is more powerful than the pleasure they might gain. Moving away from pain is a survival instinct built into our system. It is how nature ensured we'd survive on the planet. We linked pain to things that hurt us and avoided them from that moment on. So if you link pain to birth or any aspect of having a baby, you will be programming yourself away from it. If you link pleasure to motherhood, and if you change your thoughts, you will change your reality, and then you will be more likely to become pregnant and have a healthy pregnancy. Of course all women wanting a baby do link huge amounts of pleasure to imagining hearing the news that they are pregnant, but they often have other beliefs under the surface that are disrupting their ability to become and stay pregnant.

On many occasions, I have asked clients who long to be pregnant to close their eyes and imagine they have just had their pregnancy confirmed, and to tell me how they feel. They always answer, 'Oh thrilled, delighted.' But when I asked them to imagine the next feeling, one said, 'Terrified,' and another said, 'Actually, I am so scared my husband will leave me with the baby, because my first husband left me, and I had no idea I even felt that until now.' Another said, 'When my mum had my brother, I felt so left out and excluded my close relationship with her ended as soon as my brother was born. My husband is the only person in the world I have just for me, who really loves me more than anything or anyone else, and I am scared the baby might end that, and he might love the baby more than me.'

You can see how insidious these hidden, underlying beliefs are, but as long as you do the exercises I have written for you, you will be able to get rid of them.

"What the mind can conceive, the body can achieve. Visualisation can get you pregnant."

Anon.

STEP FIVE:

See My Baby

In this Step, I am going to show you how to easily and effectively programme your mind to improve your fertility. In order to be a mother, you absolutely *must* be able to see yourself as blissfully, happily pregnant, and then happily raising your child. You can do it with practice, and if you take just five minutes a day, every day, to visualise yourself as a happy, relaxed, and capable mother, you are raising your chances of becoming one. Scientists in America and Europe have proved that visualisation techniques dramatically impact our bodies. When you see yourself as pregnant, you send a clear message to your brain that affects your energy levels, your hormones, and your motivation. These changes cause physical sensations, which in turn affect your thoughts and feelings, which in turn reinforce the mental programming. Thinking positively about conception and pregnancy can activate particular neurons in the brain, which secrete hormones such as endogenous opiates, which make us feel good about ourselves. Negative thoughts have the opposite effect. Particular neurons are involved with producing negative thoughts, and they also produce negative hormones, such as cortisol, a stress hormone that leads to feelings of anxiety...one of nature's forms of birth control. While forming different pictures in your mind, you must also eliminate every possible negative word and focus only on what you wish to achieve, which is to have your baby. Keep your mind on what you want, and off what you don't want. Whatever you focus on, you will move towards, so focusing on *not* conceiving, or having a miscarriage, simply puts negative words and images back into your mind. We all have an imagination, or we would never worry, or respond to scary images on the television.

I frequently meet clients who say things like: 'I can't imagine things,' or 'I'm just no good at visualisation.' I say to them, 'That's great! You must never worry about anything, ever.' 'Oh, but I do,' they say, and I respond, 'How can you worry if you can't imagine or visualise? How do you find your car when you return to the car park if you don't have an ability to visualise where you parked it hours earlier?'

Visualisation takes practice, and it gets easier, because what the mind sees, it believes without question. What you can hold in your mind you can accomplish, and as you visualise, you will stimulate your mind and body into action.

Everyone has an imagination, and your imagination has no limits. If you think you can't see or imagine your reproductive system becoming super fertile, remember the power of thought. Thinking of it will make it happen. When you think or even hear about something, your mind always makes a picture of what that looks like. So even though you *believe* you are not able to visualise, your mind is actually seeing it in great detail; you are just not aware of it. You can see yourself as fertile, and you can see yourself enjoying being pregnant and giving birth to your perfect baby. Everything that happens is linked to how we see ourselves. You are more likely to become pregnant to the degree that you are able to see yourself as fertile. If you practice skills of visualisation and combine them with programming the subconscious mind, you will get much better results.

We have amazing potential to influence our cells, to tell them how to behave, and make them act accordingly. I always describe cells as being like schoolchildren in that they know exactly what to do and how to do it, but if they aren't working to our satisfaction, they need to be commanded, instructed, or shown what to do. What we see and believe is what we ultimately become.

Your mind already has a memory of how your body performed when you were at your most fertile, and you can manifest this just by thinking of it. This means that as you think about cells performing in a particular way, you can activate their ability to perform in that way. Think hard about swallowing, do it now, as you read this, and you will notice that you want to swallow. Your mind responds to the picture and makes you do it. Think about scratching your nose, and you will find your nose starting to itch, because what we think about, the body brings about. This happens both consciously and subconsciously, so even as you sleep, your subconscious mind is affecting your hormones. If you programme your mind correctly, you can influence your egg quality, your womb lining, your ovulation, and your whole reproductive system.

Your subconscious mind is much stronger than your conscious mind. It is said that only 10 per cent of our mind is conscious, and the other 90 per cent is subconscious, while willpower accounts for only 4 per cent of the conscious mind percentage. The conscious mind is the mind of choice, while the subconscious is the mind of preference, and we always choose what we prefer. This is important because while you may consciously long for a baby, your subconscious mind may prefer something quite different. In areas of conflict, the subconscious mind will always win because it can make the conscious do whatever it likes. This is particularly relevant in areas such as overeating, where the conscious desire may be to lose weight, but the subconscious has some deeper preference for the excess weight, often as a form of insulation or barrier. So you may have a conscious desire to be a mother, but at the same time a subconscious desire to avoid pregnancy or birth or hospitals. The subconscious desire is more likely to win, because it is more dominant and able to affect the workings of your body. Some hypochondriacs have a strong conscious desire to be well, but the subconscious desire is to be ill, because illness allows them to receive attention, including love, touch, nurturing, time and concern. So while they may wish to be well they also have a subconscious wish to be ill, which is more dominant. The subconscious is at least 90 per cent stronger than the conscious, and the subconscious mind works thirty thousand times faster than the conscious. So if you are set on making changes but think you only have to make them consciously, you will find it a harder, longer, less successful, and less lasting process than if you make those changes subconsciously.

If you want to change any behaviour, you must be absolutely sure to make changes both consciously and subconsciously. Your mind will always do what it *thinks* you want it to do, but unless you are clear when programming your mind it will do things with the right intention, but often get the wrong result.

If at any time in your past you verbalised not wanting to be pregnant your mind picked up a belief that you do not want to be pregnant. It may still believe that now and its intention is to keep you that way despite your more recent desire for a baby.

It is rather like finding that someone who came in to clean your house has moved all your things and put them back in the wrong place. That person's intention is to help you, but unless you are able to clearly state, 'Don't move the papers on my desk, and don't throw out that pile of magazines, but please do this and this,' then you won't get the result you intended. You would have got a better result if you had been clearer and more detailed in your instructions. If you go to the hairdresser and say, 'Cut my hair,' without being specific, it is not very likely that you will get the cut you want, even though the hairdresser is doing what he or she thinks you want. It is the same with your mind. If you are detailed and specific, you are more likely to get what you want, and if you are vague and unspecific, you are less likely to get what you want.

Specificity is important because your mind has no capacity to reason. It will lock onto ideas that are not specific or detailed enough or are outdated, and you won't get the results you want or could have. For instance, if someone longed for attention, he could develop a nervous habit, which would get him lots of attention, but not the kind he wanted. If you want attention, make sure you programme your subconscious by letting it know that you only want positive, beneficial attention. When children want attention, they don't care if it's positive or negative. They just want attention. Some children and adults can fall victim to a variety of illnesses because they are not getting the attention they need.

Sometimes the subconscious need or desire for attention can be so great that it can cause a person to go from one symptom of illness to another, completely overruling the conscious desire to be fit and well.

If you long for a rest because you are overworked, and say things like, 'I would love a week off just staying in bed,' and then you end up in bed with flu, it is an example of the subconscious being incorrectly programmed. If you say that you are dreading the party or meeting on Wednesday, and that you would give anything not to go, you might wake up on Wednesday with an upset stomach or severe headache that prevents you from going. Your mind thinks it has done what you wanted, and in a way, it has, but in a very ineffective and counterproductive way.

I once worked with a girl who was late for everything, causing her lots of anxiety and unhappiness. She realised whilst in hypnosis that this started as a child when she was desperate for attention and would miss the school bus so her father would have to drive her to school. As an adult, she was continuing the pattern of being late, and was attracting lots of unwanted attention, as she was a teacher and would always be the last to arrive at her own class. When she'd attend a lecture or concert, she would always be the last one to enter the room, so everyone would turn to look at her or stand up to let her pass, which she hated, but it got her a lot of attention. She was able to change this behaviour by letting her subconscious know that this practice was outdated and inappropriate, that it caused her anxiety, and had a negative effect on her career. As she told herself that she only wanted positive and beneficial attention, she ceased being late and actually started to get to places early. She was delighted with this because it made such a difference in her life. She was calmer, she did not miss trains or appointments, and she was able to develop a reputation for being punctual (although it took her friends and family a while to get used to the new behaviour.)

Your mind is the most effective and powerful tool for implementing positive changes in your life. As you follow each chapter of this book, step by step, you will become an expert at programming your subconscious mind, and you will find the more you do it, the better you become at it, and the more you enjoy it.

Remember to go to my website www.tryingtogetpregnant.co.uk to see pictures of the embryo as it develops. These images will help you picture what is going on in your womb. Look at the amazing book *A Child is Born,* by Lennart Nilsson, which has the most beautiful and detailed pictures of conception and of the developing foetus in the womb. Also of course be aware of what is going on in your body as it gets ready for conception. You have a window of opportunity to conceive every month, and it all comes down to the timing of when your egg is released. Once ovulated, an egg lives for twenty-four to thirty-six hours, whereas sperm live for a few days. If you have a twenty-eight-day cycle, you will ovulate fourteen days after the first day of your period, and if you have a thirty-two-day cycle, you will ovulate eighteen days after the first day. It's really important to have sex both before and after ovulation to maximize the likelihood of sperm and egg meeting. It is worth using an ovulation predictor kit to be certain of your ovulation dates.

You can use visualisation techniques to imagine your body releasing an egg that is of perfect quality and able to live for the longest amount of time, while giving off a powerful chemical that draws to it a perfect sperm, like a heat-seeking missile. You can buy some excellent kits that tell you when you are ovulating, and you will be able to notice changes in your body. The most obvious sign that you are ready to conceive is a slight change in the consistency of your cervical mucus. During ovulation, it changes into a thin, stretchy, and clear texture rather like egg white (you can stretch it between your fingers) and your body produces quite a lot of it. The job of this mucus is to nourish, protect, and increase the speed of the sperm as it travels to meet the egg, so the more of this changed, textured mucus there is, the more your body is ready to receive the sperm and result in pregnancy. This is the most fertile time for conception to occur. Other signs of ovulation are; your body temperature will rise after ovulation and lower abdominal discomfort or twinges can also be a sign of ovulation for one-fifth of women.

Eight steps to programming the subconscious mind for pregnancy and birth.

1: Be positive.
Eliminate every possible negative word connected to pregnancy, birth, and babies, and focus only on what you wish to achieve (a perfect pregnancy and a perfect, healthy, robust baby) and move towards it.

2: Be absolutely clear.
Keep your mind on what you want, and off what you don't want. Whatever you focus on, you will move towards, so thinking about how you *don't* want to look, feel, or become, simply puts negative words and images back into your mind. For example: 'I feel excited and positive about having a baby', *not* 'I am not scared about having a handicapped baby'. 'I am fertile and healthy', *not* 'I am not too old to get pregnant'. 'I will have a perfect and wonderful pregnancy', *not* 'I will not miscarry'.

No, *not*, and *don't* are all neutral words, and have no effect on the subconscious mind. That's why thinking the words, 'I am not sleepy, I don't feel tired,' causes the mind to lock onto the only descriptive words in the sentence, which are *tired* and *sleepy*. If you keep saying, 'I don't feel sick,' your mind is locking onto the descriptive word 'sick,' so replace it with, 'I feel wonderfully healthy.' Thinking 'I am not getting older' focuses on the only descriptive word, which is 'older,' so replace it with 'I am young and fertile.'

By turning over any negative thoughts, you will find the positive, because they are the flip side of your thinking.

3: Be specific, and use very descriptive words.
The words we use in front of words (either adjectives or adverbs) increase or decrease the effect of those words. Rather than say, 'I am fertile,' say, 'I am *extremely* fertile' or '*fantastically* fertile' *or* '*super* fertile.' Say, 'I have *abundant* energy, *massive* amounts of energy.' Instead of saying, 'I am a good parent,' change it to, 'I am a *loving, caring, wonderful, fantastic* mother.'

The mind only responds to words that are symbolic, which make a picture, so use words that are very symbolic and very descriptive. For example, 'I have abundant premium grade-A eggs. I am robustly healthy throughout my pregnancy. I am creating a healthy, robust, resilient, perfect baby. My baby's birth is exciting and thrilling and wonderful. I look and feel marvellous and radiant during my pregnancy.'

Don't worry if this all seems a little farfetched and not strictly true. Your subconscious mind has no capacity to reason and will believe whatever you tell it, especially if you tell it often enough, so you might as well go for it and exaggerate every point.

In the English language, there are four thousand words for emotions and feelings, yet many people use the same twelve words over and over to describe how they are feeling. Using different words will change your biochemistry, so when you are describing yourself, use words like *super fertile, fabulous, excellent, superbly healthy, enthusiastic, radiant, outstanding, exceptional, wonderful, young, marvellous, robustly healthy, and so on.*

4: Use the present tense.
The subconscious mind is only in the moment, so create images that are occurring now, this instant. For example, 'My eggs *are* becoming stronger, more fertile, and more resilient today and every day. My fertility *is* increasing

rapidly and progressively right now. I *am* expecting my baby now.'

Never use the word 'my' as a prefix to something you wish to be free from: *my* infertility, *my* weak womb, *my* fears, *my* weird cervix, *my* period pain, *my* nausea, *my* worries, *my* useless eggs, *my* miscarriages. This causes the mind to accept something as belonging to you when it doesn't. A good rule of the thumb is: If you don't want to keep it, don't call it *mine*. Your mind finds it much easier to change things and let go of things when it believes you don't want them, but if you call those same things *mine* it is very confusing to the mind. Remember that the mind cannot maintain conflicting beliefs, so referring to something as 'mine' while wanting to be free of it is conflicting. It soon becomes easy to say *the* worries, *the* fears, *the* anxiety, so start doing it now, and keep doing it. If you have a pain instead of saying *my* aches and pains, or *my* pain or *my* headache, change it to *the* aches and pains, *the* pain, *the* headache and so on.

If your programming says 'Next year, or even next month, I will become pregnant,' your mind cannot create a proper image of it, because your mind only works in the present tense, so you must say, 'I am becoming pregnant now.' It is very beneficial to add the words 'now' or 'right now' to the end of every statement you make: My body is becoming super fertile *right now.* I am enjoying a radiant pregnancy *now.* I am ovulating the most perfect eggs right *now.* My baby is powerfully connected to me right *now.* My baby is growing perfectly within me *now.* My fertilised egg is implanting and attaching securely in my womb *now.*

5: Be detailed.
Make your words dynamic and descriptive: 'I am young, vibrantly healthy, and fertile, with grade-A perfect abundant eggs.' Make it personal: '*I* am,' *I* look,' '*I* always,' '*I* can.'

6: Visualisation must be vivid.
See it, sense it, feel it, touch it, and hear it. Activate all your senses, because the more vividly you visualise, the more rapidly your mind responds.

Feel the sensation of carrying your baby through a full-term, healthy, wonderful pregnancy. *Feel* your baby kicking as it becomes stronger. *Feel* the emotion and delight of giving birth to a perfect baby.

See your new-born in your arms, *feel* yourself holding your baby in your arms *touching* its perfect skin and downy hair, *feeling* its tiny hand gripping your finger. *Imagine* touching your baby's skin, *feeling* how soft and satiny it is, *touching* its toes and fingers, *stroking* your baby, patting and rocking instinctively. *Sense* your body responding to your instructions, so you give birth easily and nurse your baby with ease. *Hear* your baby *gurgling, listen* to it breathing, *and love* hearing those baby sounds. *Smell* that lovely baby smell. *Taste* it as you kiss and nuzzle your baby. *Feel* the weight of your baby in your arms. *Feel* its warm body heat, *hear* its heartbeat, so strong and rhythmic.

7: Visualisation must be frequent.
The more vividly you visualise, the more rapidly your mind and body respond. Visualise frequently, and repeat it over and over, like playing a video in your head. Repetition is vital. When you repeat an action, you create a neural pathway in your brain that is strengthened with each repetition. This pathway is like a thread that becomes stronger every time you repeat something, until it becomes more like a cable. When you first learnt to use a keyboard, drive a car, or operate a new mobile phone, you had to repeat the actions slowly. Now, due to repetition, they are so embedded in you they are almost automatic.

8: Use duration and intensity.

Hold the picture for longer and make it bigger, brighter, and clearer. Combine your visualisation with an intensity of desire, as this will increase the effectiveness. Visualisation takes practice. What the mind sees, it believes without question, so your ability to visualise will have a powerful effect on you. As you visualise you will stimulate your mind and body into action. Remember, what you can hold in your mind with confidence and feeling, you can achieve. Become much clearer about what you want. The more you visualise, the more you will believe your visualisation is possible. Successful people visualise all the time. We can all change our thinking and the mental pictures we make, and as we improve them, we can improve everything. By changing your thinking and your focus, and by making changes in the language you use, you can increase your fertility.

If you think you can't do it, be aware that you are already visualising that outcome all the time. Every time you say 'I can't get pregnant; it doesn't work for me; it's impossible for me to conceive; I am just too old; my eggs are past it,' you are already visualising a specific result, and it's working.

You might as well use good visualisations, as your mind will believe and act on whatever you tell it (good or bad) because your mind responds to the pictures you make in your head and the words you say to yourself.

Baby Exercises: 7.

You are now ready to make a programme tailored specifically for you. Go through the following eight steps, and write out a plan. By step eight, your thoughts will have become one or more paragraphs.

Begin now by taking a thought such as 'I am super fertile' and writing it out as number one.

1: *I am super fertile.*

2: Go to step two, and decide how you can be absolutely crystal clear about fact number one, and write it down.

3: Now increase your sentence into a paragraph, using very descriptive words and keeping it all in the present tense: *I am super fertile because I am so connected to the life force of my baby and because I am directing my body to increase my fertility, and my body is responding perfectly.*

4: Make it even more personal. This is all about you, as you want to be, so add more words and thoughts. Put powerful positive words in front of your sentences: *I am amazingly fertile. I have superb and excellent eggs. My body is... I have the energy level of...* and so on. Use several thoughts and then connect them in a statement as you work through this exercise, so the end result will leave you with an exciting, easy-to-memorise statement about yourself rather than several lines of short sentences.

5: Make it even more detailed by adding in: *I am... I always... I feel... I can... I look... I have... I carry...* to your programme.

6: Use and activate all your senses by adding in the words *feel, sense, touch, see, hear, imagine.*

7: Keep working on it until you have it exactly as you want it. Then read it and repeat it to yourself over and over until it becomes embedded in your mind. This will happen quite quickly and easily. Your programme should not be so long that you can't recall it, or so short that it does not make enough impact on your mind.

8: Now you are ready to close your eyes and begin to imagine what you have created and chosen for yourself. Again, it really doesn't matter if you don't seem to make vivid pictures. By now your mind is absolutely responding to the words and images, whether you are seeing them clearly or not.

A finished example of this could be:
'I am conceiving my baby by thinking about my fertility and seeing my healthy egg moving into my womb, attracting to it the healthiest sperm by giving off a powerful chemical that draws the sperm to it. Fertilisation, conception, and impregnation takes place. My baby is growing in me, and I am influencing it in the most positive way throughout my perfect pregnancy. I have a belief system that allows me to believe and know this is possible. I have excellent fertility. My eggs are compatible with my partner's sperm. I have such a strong desire and belief in my ability to have a baby. My baby is moving into my womb and into my life right now.'
OR
'I ovulate the most perfect grade-A premium egg that draws to it the most perfect sperm. My egg is fertilised, and conception and pregnancy begins as my fertilised egg moves into my womb and attaches and grows securely there. I am expecting a baby. I am a mother to be. My body is fertile and healthy. It is nurturing and supporting my developing baby. I am so connected to my baby, and my baby is so connected to me. It stays in my healthy womb and grows strong and perfect. My

womb is designed to carry my baby to full term, so my womb does a superb job of nurturing and growing my strong, robust baby. While my body nourishes my baby physically, I nourish it emotionally. My baby feels so loved and wanted. It has a strong life force, and it stays with me throughout my perfect pregnancy.'

When we hold a thought, plan, goal, or idea continuously in our mind our subconscious works to bring it to a reality. Many of my clients tell me they don't believe this, because they have had a plan in their minds that has never come to fruition. This is always because they have not done the groundwork. They have not cleared their mind of conflicting thoughts and beliefs beforehand, and although they may have a plan in their minds, they have not programmed their minds in a specific way that will allow the plan to be realised.

If you follow the detailed and specific steps designed to allow you to programme your mind for success, you can succeed. You can continue to hold your programme in your mind by writing and rewriting it, reviewing it, talking about it, and visualising it. Some people are very visual and respond to how things look, while others respond better to how things sound or feel. This is known as being auditory, visual or kinaesthetic, and whichever you tend to be, this programme will work for you.

People who respond most instinctively to how things look are known as visual. People who respond to how things feel are known as kinaesthetic, and people who respond to how things sound are known as auditory. It is possible to be a combination of all three or to be predominantly one with aspects of the others. If you know that you are mostly visual, focus more of your programme on how you look pregnant, and what your baby looks like. Imagine seeing your positive pregnancy test and your home filled with baby things...the cot, the pram in the hall, the car seat in the car, the sandpit in the garden, the highchair in the kitchen, the baby bath and lotions in your bathroom and baby toys in your lounge. See yourself coming home from hospital with your baby in your arms to a house full of cards, flowers, balloons, gifts, and visitors longing to meet your baby.

If you are more kinaesthetic, focus more on how you feel carrying your baby inside you, and loving the different sensations as your baby grows in you for nine months. Focus on feeling euphoric as you give birth, then feeling like a natural, competent mother feeding your new-born with ease. Focus on the feeling of holding your baby in your arms and feeling its warmth. Imagine feeling so good as you take your baby home and feeling so proud and complete when your friends and family come to visit you and your baby.

If you are predominantly auditory, you can focus on hearing your doctor confirming the news that you are pregnant and hearing all the congratulations from your family as you announce you are having a baby. Hear your doctor at every visit telling you that your pregnancy is progressing in a textbook perfect way; hear your baby's sounds as it is born, hear the heartbeat on the scan, and so on.

A combination of all three is fine, and you will find some prewritten scripts in the next Step for conception, perfect pregnancy, and birth, so you can choose one of these if you prefer. You have the option of pre-recorded CDs and downloads for conception, IVF conception, pregnancy, and birth. You also have the option of contacting us via www.tryingtogetpregnant.co.uk and we will make a programme for you.

Get into the habit of reading and repeating your programme to yourself prior to falling asleep. You may find it helps you to record your programme and to play it back to yourself so that you can absorb the words rather than trying to remember them, although this is not essential, because the more you look at this programme, the more your mind will retain it. You will find you can remember the programme by focusing on it and reading it until it quickly becomes embedded in your mind. It is also worth writing out the programme and pinning it to your desk, your fridge, or your mirror, or writing it out on your phone or your computer. You might also keep a copy in your wallet.

"By doing just a little more than is necessary you can achieve a great deal more than you otherwise would have."

Anon.

STEP SIX:

Baby Love

Perfect Conception
Perfect IVF Conception
Perfect Easy Pregnancy
Perfect Easy Birth

We are going to go over some varied scripts covering conception, pregnancy, and birth. You will get used to your own personal programme. The difference between your programme and these scripts is that your programme is something created just for you. It should be short, just a few paragraphs, and easy to memorise so that you can think about it and repeat it to yourself regularly at any time. These scripts are longer and more detailed. They contain more biological information and more biological terminology, and they are designed to be spoken in the third person. You can read a script to yourself each night before sleeping, so that your mind will lock onto the words.

Trying to get Pregnant (and Succeeding)

It is fine to read it to yourself in the third person, so you are saying 'you' rather than 'I.' If it feels unfamiliar, that's okay, you will soon get used to it. The most important thing to know is that you are using a highly successful technique of communicating with your body...one that gets results.

You need to read the 'conception script' for at least a month, and then once or twice a week, to condition your mind to these new beliefs and to imprint them into your memory. On average, it takes the mind twenty-one days to imprint and accept new habits and beliefs, and erase old ones.

You need to read the 'perfect pregnancy' script throughout your pregnancy, once or twice a week, and with the 'birth script,' it is ideal to have a copy of the CD or download, so you can use it daily in the last two months of your pregnancy. The scripts are written out for you exactly as they need to be read or recorded, so you will find this easy to follow.

As you take in the words, your subconscious mind will be fully accessed and receptive to the commands and mental instructions contained within each script, and will accept the suggestions more easily. When listening to these scripts, it is important to know that you don't need to be a biochemist with a perfect knowledge of the workings of your body to get results. I do have clients who say to me, 'When I listen to your CD, I don't understand some of the descriptions or phrases. Does that mean I won't get such good results?' You can get great results whether you understand the wording or not, because your body understands the descriptions completely and perfectly and will do the work for you. All you need to do is believe it will work, expect it to work, and expect to get great results.

Most people, when asked to place their hands on their stomach, will put their hands below their navel and over their intestines. In fact, the stomach is actually above the navel, under the ribs and above the waist. The inability to correctly place where your stomach sits does not stop it from working. You don't need a full knowledge of how your body works to get results, because knowledge of the mind-body connection in making changes is more beneficial to you than a biological understanding of your body. However, you do need to know when you ovulate, as some women only have one day in the month when they can conceive, and missing that day or having too much sex beforehand can mean not enough good quality sperm is left.

If your doctor said to you, 'You have an inflamed pituitary gland' or 'You have a problem with your cranium,' you might be in the dark in terms of locating those body parts, but your mind can manifest the symptoms that match the diagnosis, despite the fact that you are not consciously visualising them because you don't understand the language or medical jargon. In the same way children can hear a parent say, 'I have irritable bowel syndrome' or 'I have migraine,' and although the children don't understand these words, they can still develop similar symptoms, because they mirror their parents, without understanding anything about biology.

From the list of scripts below, choose one that is relevant to you, and listen to it or read it every day until your mind is absolutely familiar with it. The 'IVF script' has been designed to be played throughout each IVF procedure. You can of course choose just to play the relevant CD or download every day, but it is still a good idea to read the scripts through to become familiar with them.

1: Conception.
Your inner mind, the most powerful part of you, is locking on to these words and accepting them easily. Your mind's job is to do what it thinks you want it to do, so you are letting your mind know with precision, accuracy, and clarity

that what you want and insist on is to conceive your perfect baby. Your mind is becoming more and more aware that you have a strong desire and a powerful motivation and ability to conceive your baby, to become pregnant, and to have a child.

You are now ready and able to motivate your reproductive system to act as a young, perfect reproductive system. You have the power to influence your body to communicate with your womb, ovaries, and eggs, and to have them respond to your instructions.

You are now using the power of your mind to direct and command your body to become super fertile. Because your body is controlled by a network of intelligence, which is influenced by your mind, you are able to relax deeply enough to influence your own mind and to improve your fertility.

You accept only positive ideas about your fertility and imprint them onto your body. You are communicating with the intelligence of your reproductive system and responding to these words as you think about becoming a mother.

When you were younger, you were super fertile. Your body has a memory of this, and you are reactivating it just by thinking of it. You are activating this memory and increasing your fertility just by thinking these thoughts and hearing these words. Think of your womb lining as perfect. Your hormone levels are perfect for pregnancy. Your eggs are young, strong and healthy. Imagine and feel your body getting ready for a perfect pregnancy. Everything is performing more effectively every time you think these thoughts.

Everything is in the right place at the right time to ensure you conceive. Your thoughts are commanding your body to perform at peak fertility, as it did in your youth. Whatever you focus on, you move towards. You ovulate the most perfect grade-A premium egg, which is fertilised and then nourished and nurtured by your body as it develops into your baby. Your thoughts are so powerful that they are creating physical changes in your body right now.

As you relax and take in these words, know that your mind responds to your thinking, to the words and images you make.

See your eggs as resilient and plentiful. Rehearse with your egg what it has to do. See it moving into the fallopian tube, drawing to it a perfect sperm and becoming fertilised, then moving into your womb and securely attaching itself there, knowing that it belongs there, that this is its happy home for the next nine months. Your embryo recognises your womb as home and secures itself. Like a plant with long, strong roots, it firmly implants itself into your womb, where it grows perfectly on target for the next nine months. Your baby grows safely and securely and you do a wonderful job of growing and developing your baby perfectly. Your mind is influencing your body, and you are influencing your mind in the most perfect way. You are developing a clear mental image, where you see yourself conceiving and carrying your baby to full term, knowing the more you see it, the more rapidly it will occur.

Your ability to think these thoughts, to see these images, and to accept these suggestions, is having a powerful effect on your fertility right now. You are able to stimulate your mind which in turn stimulates your body and just hearing these words is causing your inner mind to picture it and create it perfectly. Your imagination has no limits. You see your baby, and as you do, you are reinforcing your subconscious mind, and replacing negative thoughts with new positive ones. As you focus on achieving motherhood, with confidence in your ability to make it happen, you can achieve it.

This image of you as a mother is becoming more real, more attainable, and clearer, each time you hear this script. Your inner mind (the most powerful part of you) is locking on to these words, hearing them over and over again, and they are becoming a powerful part of your memory. See your home full of baby things. Your baby's presence is everywhere, and you like it that way. Talk to your baby, and let it know how much you love it, how much you want it. Know that what you want, wants you, and what you are moving towards is moving towards you, until the moment you are delivering your baby.

2: IVF Conception.

Your inner mind (the most powerful part of you) is locking onto these words and accepting them easily. Your mind's job is to do what it thinks you want it to do, so you are letting your mind know with precision, accuracy, and clarity that what you want and insist on is to respond to your IVF treatment perfectly, so that the end result is you as a mother, carrying and delivering your healthy baby. The IVF is a perfect success for you. You ovulate plenty of healthy grade-A eggs that respond perfectly to fertilisation. Your eggs are strong and robust and compatible with your partner's sperm. They develop perfectly, and at the embryo transfer, the right embryo attaches and takes, and grows, over nine months, into your perfect baby.

Your IVF is 100 per cent successful at every stage. You achieve 100 per cent success at egg collection and 100 per cent success at fertilisation, and 100 per cent success at the embryo transfer, where your embryo recognises your womb as home and securely implants into your womb. Like a plant with long, strong roots, it firmly attaches itself to your womb, where it grows perfectly on target for the next nine months. You conceive your perfect baby. Your mind is focused on your strong desire and powerful ability to conceive your baby, to become pregnant, and to have a child.

During your IVF, you welcome every procedure and every drug, and every injection is taking you closer to your baby.

While you are lying in the clinic, you take your mind to nine months ahead, where you are lying in another clinic delivering your perfect baby. This image always thrills and delights you and motivates your body to be happy and welcoming towards every step of your IVF. You are now ready and able to motivate your reproductive system to act as a young, perfect reproductive system. You have the power to influence your body to communicate with your womb, ovaries, and eggs, and to have them respond to your instructions. As soon as your embryo is transferred back into your body, you talk to it. You tell it to attach, to grow, to love being in such a warm, safe, loving place.

You direct and command your body to respond perfectly to every step of IVF. Your body is controlled by a network of intelligence, which is influenced by your mind. You are able to relax deeply enough to influence your body to welcome the IVF and to have it be 100 per cent successful. You accept only positive ideas about your response to IVF, and imprint them onto your body. You are communicating with the intelligence of your reproductive system and responding to these words as you think about becoming a mother.

Your womb lining and your FSH levels are perfect. Your hormone levels are perfect for pregnancy. Your eggs are young and healthy. Your body is ready for your perfect pregnancy. Everything is performing more effectively every time you think these thoughts. Everything is in the right place at the right time to ensure you conceive, and your body is working at peak fertility, as it did in your youth. You ovulate the most perfect grade-A premium eggs, which are fertilised, and then nourished and nurtured by your body as it develops your baby. Your thoughts are so powerful that they help your body to respond perfectly to IVF.

As you relax and take in these words, your mind responds to your thoughts, words, and images. See your eggs as resilient and plentiful at egg collection, being fertilised by perfect sperm, and developing perfectly at every stage. The right embryo is transferred into your womb, and securely and firmly attaches to your womb, knowing it belongs there, that this is its happy home for the next nine months. Your womb does a wonderful job of growing and developing your baby perfectly. Your mind is influencing your body, and you are influencing your mind in the most perfect way. You are developing a clear mental image, seeing yourself conceiving and carrying your baby to full term, knowing the more you see it, the more rapidly it will occur.

Your ability to think these thoughts, to see these images, and to accept these suggestions, is having a powerful effect on your fertility right now. Just thinking of it is causing your inner mind to picture it and manifest it perfectly. Your imagination has no limits. You see your baby, and as you do, you are reinforcing your subconscious mind, replacing negative thoughts with new positive ones, as you focus on achieving motherhood with confidence in your ability to make it happen. You can achieve it. This image of you as a mother is becoming more real, more attainable, and clearer, each time you hear this script. Your inner mind (the most powerful part of you) is locking onto these words, hearing them over and over again, as they become a powerful part of your memory. See your home full of baby things. Your baby's presence is everywhere, and you like it that way. Talk to your baby, and let it know how much you love it, how much you want it. Know that what you want wants you and what you are moving towards is moving towards you, until the moment you are delivering your baby.

3: Perfect Pregnancy.
Your body has made a perfect baby, and it is now growing, nurturing, and nourishing your baby through your perfect

pregnancy. Your body is so intelligent, it made a baby, and it can now grow and develop your baby without any help from you at all, but you love being involved in your baby's development, so you talk to it every day, and as your body does a perfect job of physically growing your baby, you do a perfect job of emotionally developing and nurturing your baby. You have a deep emotional attachment to your baby. It knows it is much loved and wanted, and it grows strong and resilient every day. You tell your baby at every stage what it is doing, and every part of your baby develops on target. Its heart and lungs are strong. Its immune system and central nervous system are perfect. Its skeletal system is perfect. Its hands and fingers and toes, its eyes, mouth, and ears…every part of your baby grows perfectly, as in a textbook pregnancy. Your body and baby are working as a perfect team. You and your body are working as a perfect team. You and your baby are a perfect team. Your baby is powerfully and safely connected to you and to your body. It knows how much you love it and how much you have to offer it, and it grows every day. You can see your bump at twelve weeks, at twenty-five weeks, and at forty weeks. Your body is showing your resilient baby bump. You love looking radiantly pregnant, and every day you focus on your healthy baby growing inside you, getting ready to be born to you safely and well at the end of your happy, perfect pregnancy.

4: Easy Happy Birth.
Your body has carried your baby to full term and done a perfect job of growing a healthy, strong baby, and just as your body knew how to make and grow your baby, it also knows exactly how to deliver it. You feel reassured that your body knows how to deliver your baby, and when the time is right your baby gets into position in the birth canal. It moves, and at the same time your body begins the birth process. The round muscles that have held your

baby safely in place relax to let the baby move out of your body, and as the round muscles relax, the long muscles contract to push your baby out of your body. This works in perfect sequence. The long muscles contract, and the stronger these contractions are, the closer your baby is to being born. You welcome every contraction. You breathe deeply. You talk to your baby. You tell it to hurry up and move out of your body and into your arms, as you can't wait to hold it. Your baby picks up your message, and it swiftly moves down the birth canal. Your skin stretches easily. Your babies head crowns, and you can put your hands down and feel the top of your baby's head. You are ready to push. You are wonderful at birth, pushing when you need to, breathing in between contractions, and delivering your baby into an atmosphere of joy and delight and calmness. You push out your baby's head, and then with one more push, you have delivered your baby. You deliver the afterbirth, and you are holding your baby in your arms. You are a natural mother. You instinctively know how to pat and soothe and rock your baby. You give birth so easily. Your baby's birth is a wonderful day for you. It's one of the best days of your life, and because you are so calm, so happy, so strong, and positive, you deliver a happy, calm baby that is deeply connected to you. You are so proud that you made this baby and delivered it so easily. Your birth experience, your baby's birthday, is a wonderful day for you and for your baby.

"Man is made by his belief. As he believes, so he is."

Johann Wolfgang von Goethe.

STEP SEVEN:

Baby Goals and Affirmations

Affirmations are statements of truth. Here, an affirmation is simply a short statement you repeat to yourself over and over for a few minutes daily. It might be something like: 'I am expecting a baby' or 'I am a mother-to-be' or 'My baby is coming into my life now.'

Repeat the affirmation over and over, out loud to yourself, to allow your subconscious mind to accept it. It won't always happen instantly, because we often pick an affirmation that can conflict with some beliefs we may have. One of the reasons we are covering affirmations at this point is because by now you will have changed some beliefs and will be open to the idea of changing more.

Many people give up with affirmations because their mind seems to have so many objections to them. They don't really believe what they are saying, or understand that there is a system for making the mind accept and believe affirmations, so they find the process frustrating and abandon it.

I have found the best way to overcome this is to write out each affirmation as a statement, and just notice any objections that come to mind. Then write out the objections your mind comes up with. Keep on writing out the affirmation, with any objections or thoughts that come to mind directly underneath in your notebook.

It is important not to spend time attempting to analyse or rationalise the objections. Just write them out and keep going so that you write down each affirmation and any objection or response.

As you look over the statement and the objections you have written, you may notice a distinct pattern emerging, because the more you keep writing out the affirmation, the fewer objections your mind will come up with. Eventually your mind will exhaust the objections, and it will simply say, *'Okay, I agree, I accept it. You are expecting a baby.'*

Here is an example: The chosen affirmation is: *I am a mother-to-be.*

Your mind may immediately come up with some objections, especially if you have been conditioned by old beliefs. They may be things like: *I am too old. It is not possible for me. I have tried for years, and nothing has worked. I always miscarry. Everyone will laugh at me if I do this. This is all rubbish. My eggs are useless. I don't believe in this. Actually I do believe in this a little. I will make myself believe in this. There are examples of women like me having a baby. If other people can do it, so can I. Okay, it's true, I can have a baby.*

As you continue to write out each affirmation, and say it out loud, your objections will become weaker and weaker. You will pay them less and less attention. Your belief in your affirmation will become stronger. Eventually your mind will run out of objections and will fully accept the affirmation. Get into the habit of repeating your affirmations daily, and make sure you say them out loud. It doesn't matter if you feel silly; most people do initially. Just become aware of how you feel and the thoughts and feelings you experience as you say each affirmation. It's good to repeat your affirmations at night just before you go to sleep, and again in the morning just after waking, when your subconscious is most receptive. It is also a very good idea to write out your affirmations and to pin them up on a mirror or the fridge door, to put them in your purse or your desk, on your screen saver or your phone, and anywhere else that causes you to remind yourself of them regularly and frequently. By doing this you will be able to make your ability to have a baby an on-going affirmation.

You will develop more and more potential through the use of your affirmations, because the words and images you repeat over and over to yourself become the blueprint for who you become. Positive affirmations go into the subconscious and eventually replace negative thoughts. The subconscious responds best to clear, authoritative commands. The clearer, more precise and straightforward they are, the more rapidly the mind accepts them and begins to work on them.

Affirmations can also build self-esteem, turn you into an optimist, and diminish negative self-talk. So please make sure you write out your affirmations in your notebook using the instructions in this Step. Write out every objection you come up with until you have exhausted the objections. Then look at what you have written and what you can learn from that.

Baby Goals

Goals and goal setting for motherhood

Many tests over many years, including several done at Harvard, Yale, and Cornell Universities, as well as the famous Maslow tests, show that people who set goals are always the happiest and have a very high tendency to achieve their goals.

Think about *your* goals. When you bought this book, you had the goal of having your baby. At this stage in the book, you have already made some changes that have increased your ability to achieve that goal. Having a goal and taking steps to accomplish it, seems to fire within us a stronger ability to reach that goal. In 1979 members of the MBA graduating programme at Harvard were asked, 'Have you set clear, written goals for your future and made plans to accomplish them?' Only 3 per cent had done it; 13 per cent had goals that were not written out, and 84 per cent had no goals at all. Ten years later, the class was interviewed again. The results showed that the 3 per cent who had clear, written goals were earning ten times as much as the other 97 per cent were earning *collectively.* Even the 13 per cent who had unwritten goals were earning twice as much as the 84 per cent who had no goals. That Harvard study was a copy of a study done in 1953 at Yale University, where the graduating year was asked a series of questions, including, 'Do you have clear, specific goals written out, with plans to accomplish them? Just 3 per cent said yes. Twenty years later, they went back and interviewed the class members again and found that the 3 per cent with written goals were worth more financially than the other 97 per cent put together. Not only were they dramatically richer, they were also happier, better adjusted, and more successful at everything they did. That is the incredible power of habitually and systematically setting goals. You must write out your goals, think about your goals, talk about your goals, and make plans to achieve them, so your subconscious mind works to make your goals come to fruition. Current studies still show that less than 3 per cent of people have clear goals, and less than 1 per cent ever write them out properly. If you want to have a baby, write it out as a goal in the specific format contained further along in this Step. When you programme your goals into your brain, you move towards accomplishing them much more easily.

Of course you need to do more than simply write out your goals as if they were a wish list. You need self-discipline, determination, self-confidence, and the self-belief to stay with them until you accomplish them. Don't give up just because they don't work out the first time or as quickly as you would like them to. With your goal to have a baby, you need tenacity and a desire to keep going, and the ability to recognise that a delay is not a denial; it's simply a delay. You can't give up if things don't work out. One of my clients had six attempts at IVF and was devastated each time it didn't work, but she was determined, so she changed her doctor and her clinic. She discovered that she had an incompatibility with her husband's sperm, which the new clinic was able to work around, and she went onto have three children in three years. She would have missed out on those delightful children had she not been tenacious and determined. Louis Pasteur said, *'Let me tell you the secret that has led me to my goal; my strength today lies solely in my tenacity.'*

It's hard to understand why more people aren't encouraged to set goals and why it is not taught in schools, especially since schools that have experimented with goal setting find that children like it and benefit hugely from it.

People don't set goals, because they don't understand their importance. They don't know how, because goal setting is not taught in schools. They fear rejection, ridicule, or criticism, so they hold back from goal setting. They might fear failure, without understanding that you can't succeed without failure. The only sure way to fail is when you fail to try.

As you write out your goal of being a parent and your plan for reaching this goal, you are already taking action that moves you closer to achieving it, because your mind works in such a way that whatever you focus on, you move towards. Your subconscious mind is a natural goal-seeking device programmed to move you towards what it is you are focusing on. By focusing on your goals (especially as you write them out) you cannot help but activate the mechanism within yourself that moves you towards achieving them, because goals seem to trigger the success mechanism within us. Medical tests have shown that people who have a goal to stay alive can even defy dying, and numerous patients who have been close to death have literally postponed death until an important event, such as a birthday, a daughter's wedding, a birth in the family, or other significant date has passed. They have a goal to live until then, and tend to reach that goal.

In China they have an annual day when elders are celebrated. It's a big event that older people look forward to the way children look forward to Christmas. More elderly people die directly after this date than at any other time of year, because the goal they have is to live until this day, and to enjoy the celebration one more time. It will literally keep them alive, against the odds, until the goal has been realised.

As you think about your goal of making, carrying, and raising your child, you are already beginning to excite your imagination. As you write out your goal, immediately your conscious mind accepts that goal, while your subconscious mind goes to work to help to turn the goal into a reality. It has been stated in various studies that with goals, we have purpose and direction, because our mind

Baby Goals and Affirmations

is a goal-seeking mechanism, whereas without goals we drift and flounder. The fact that goals give us purpose, direction, and energy may explain why all successful people have goals and actively set goals for themselves. Goal setting is a very important and extremely easy skill that boasts excellent results. Many of us have no idea how important goal setting is and miss out on its benefits.

As you set your goals, remember that *what the mind can conceive and believe the mind can achieve.* Your mind takes everything you say as a command, so make your goals absolutely clear. Make sure there is no room whatsoever for misinterpretation. If you instructed a decorator to decorate your house and then left them to it, they would do what they thought you wanted, but would probably misinterpret your desires and give you a result you were not happy with. So think of your mind as a super-efficient assistant. Let it know exactly what you want, and you are far more likely to get exactly what you want. You must be ready to learn new ways of thinking, behaving, talking, and reacting. You must create a goal that is detailed, and you must write it all out clearly, so follow these steps to become successful at goal setting and achieving.

1: Set your goal.
An example could be: *I am going to conceive, carry, and deliver a perfect baby.*

2: Form a clear image of it.
Vision is vital to goal achieving. See it and visualise it as if it were already in existence. When Mark Victor Hanson wanted his book, *Chicken Soup for the Soul* to be a bestseller, he cut out the *New York Times* bestseller book list, Tippexed out the number-one entry, and typed *Chicken Soup for the Soul* in its place. Then he stuck it on

his bathroom mirror and looked at it every day. By doing this, he was visualising it, and having struggled to get his book published, and then really struggling to make it sell, it went on to be a phenomenal bestseller. The more you visualise, the more you believe, the more it is possible. Really successful people visualise all the time.

3: Commit it to paper.
Write out your goal in detail, so your subconscious mind has a clear image of what you want. Also write out all the things you are going to do to achieve your goal, from playing your CD/download and talking to your baby daily, to eating more healthy food, planning your nursery, and buying a little something as a mark of your faith that you will have a baby.

4: Get into the habit of looking at your goal every day.
Place your written goal somewhere you will always see it, and remember as you repeat this goal to yourself, your inner resources are already beginning to move towards it.

5: Write out the reasons you have for wanting to achieve this goal.
The more reasons you come up with, the more you will excite your imagination, and the more you will believe it is attainable.

6: See your goals.
Believe in them, and make your mind concentrate on them. Play them back to yourself like a video, as if they were already in existence. Do this just before you go to sleep.

7: Find a role model.

You might want to find a picture of someone who is a great role model for you, someone like Patricia Hodge, who had unexplained infertility for thirteen years but went on to have two children in her forties. Stick the picture next to your written goal so that you look at this image daily along with your goal statement. Or alter a picture of yourself, so you look visibly pregnant or are holding a new-born. Look at it every day.

8: Be tenacious.

Tenacity, stoicism, persistence, and determination are vital. Even your most important goal will not work if you give up too soon, so be persistent. Persistence is a measure of your faith in yourself and in your ability to make it succeed.

"It is by making a small difference, again and again, that you realise what an enormous difference you can make."

Anon.

STEP EIGHT:

Baby Food

There are some foods to avoid if you want to conceive, and others that you should eat regularly. An organic diet free from additives, preservatives, and chemicals (especially artificial sweetener) can boost fertility. In the West, our food is grown in soil that lacks in nutrients, so we don't get the correct amount of vitamins and minerals that we need. In addition, the preservatives and additives in most processed and refined food can upset blood sugar levels and disrupt the body's hormone balance, leading to an increase of oestrogen, which affects women's chances of conceiving. Our modern diet is far too high in starch, sugar, and carbohydrates. Refined carbohydrates can affect fertility, because the pesticides and chemicals in flour and its by-products (bread, pasta, cereals, and pastries) can be disruptive to your body. The trans-fats used in baked goods and convenience foods can also disrupt the body, because when we eat too many toxins our body has to store those toxins in fat cells, and this increase in both fat and toxins can lower your fertility. Polycystic ovary syndrome, which is a common cause of infertility and irregular and painful periods, is caused by insulin resistance or pre-diabetes. When we eat too many carbs, our insulin levels rise. You can minimise and even reverse polycystic ovary syndrome by eliminating refined carbohydrates from your diet while increasing your protein levels and cutting down on other forms of carbohydrates, including fruit juice, bread, pasta, rice, and potatoes, which are too starchy and sugary and cause sugar levels to rise when eaten freely. Sugar can interfere with your hormone levels. Highly processed carbohydrates and sugary foods can quadruple the risks of birth defects of obese pregnant women. Pregnant women who eat a lot of: corn flakes, white bread, white rice, or chocolate biscuits, put their babies at higher risk of abnormalities. Recent tests compared the diets of 454 mothers who had babies with birth defects against 462 women with healthy babies. The risk of birth defects had increased fourfold in women who ate high levels of sugar and highly refined carbohydrates, like potatoes, chocolate biscuits, and breakfast cereals. Researchers believe the high level of glucose these foods release, quickly giving a massive sugar rush followed by a rapid lowering of sugar levels, may overwhelm the baby in the womb, interfering with key development stages.

In the last few months, fruit juice, dried fruit, and excessive amounts of fruit have received a lot of bad press, because our bodies are simply not designed to cope with a lot of sugar, and it again raises insulin levels and has a negative effect on our health.

Dr Gary Shaw, from the University of California Birth Defects Monitoring Programme, states, *"There is an association between neural tube defect risk and the glycaemic index of the mothers. The risk doubles in women eating a high GI diet in pregnancy. In obese pregnant women, eating a high GI diet, the risk quadruples."* (These studies are reported in the *American Journal of Clinical Nutrition*.)

More recent studies have linked milk with infertility, as it can upset a woman's hormone balance. Milk is a growth

Baby Food

hormone, which encourages high cell growth, enabling a calf to grow rapidly so it becomes the size of its parent within months. If you eat too much dairy produce, it may lead to hormone imbalances. Milk was not designed for human consumption. It is breast milk for a calf, so if you have problems conceiving, eliminate cow's milk, and use rice, oat, or almond milk instead. You will only really miss milk in tea and coffee, and you should cut down on that too and have herb teas instead. Just two cups of coffee daily can reduce fertility by 50 per cent.[11] Caffeine is a stimulant that upsets the body's blood sugar levels and has been linked to miscarriage. Cut out cheese and butter, and use olive oil instead. Look for organic feta and halloumi cheeses (made from goat's and sheep's milk) as these do not impact your hormones in the same way as cheeses made from cow's milk. If you have any dairy produce, try to have organic as much as possible. Dairy cattle, which are not organically raised, are given antibiotics and growth hormones as part of their regular feed, which you are ingesting second-hand, and these can disrupt and upset your own hormones. All animal hormones can affect your own hormone balance. Organic produce contains significantly fewer animal and synthetic hormones.

Sperm perform best in alkaline conditions, so make sure your diet is not too acidic. Good quality protein is essential for conception, and you need to eat enough protein in the form of organic eggs, chicken, fish, lean meat, lentils, nuts, and seeds. The body can't store protein; it is a required building food, so eat it regularly during conception, pregnancy, and whilst breast-feeding.

---

11 http://healthland.time.com/2011/06/01/could-coffee-prevent-pregnancy/
http://www.midlandfertility.com/investigations-and-treatments/preparing-for-treatment/lifestyle-bmi-and-fertility
http://edition.presstv.ir/detail/63120.html
http://infertility.about.com/od/researchandstudies/a/caffeine_fertility.htm

Trying to get Pregnant (and Succeeding)

Pay attention to the type and amount of protein in your diet. You don't need a lot, but you do need it regularly. If you are a vegan and having problems conceiving, you may need to rethink your diet, at least until you have had your baby. A vegan diet can be low in, or fully lack, B vitamins, which decrease the risk of birth defects. B vitamins are very important for conception and during pregnancy, but as their greatest source is found in animal products, most vegans miss out on them (although Marmite does contain B vitamins). No matter how noble it is to be a vegan, vegetable sources of protein, with the exception of nuts and seeds are not as beneficial as animal forms of protein.

The Food Standards Agency recommends that large fish, like tuna, marlin, and swordfish should never be eaten by women intending to become pregnant. These fish live for a long time and eat smaller fish that have the highest levels of mercury. Mercury is a common pollutant in the world's oceans, and it builds up in the fish that swim there. Farm-raised salmon contain higher levels of toxins (called polychlorinated biphenyls, or PCBs) which are proven to have a negative effect on fertility. Replace these with oily fish, like mackerel, wild salmon, and sardines. You should eat these at least twice a week as part of your pre-conception diet as well as when you are pregnant. You can also take selenium, which prevents the body from absorbing mercury, so it is advisable if you eat a diet high in all types of fish.

Many of the foods you eat daily, and assume are harmless, could be affecting and limiting your ability to conceive. For instance a breakfast of coffee with milk, cereal with milk and white toast with jam can disrupt your fertility. Don't see avoiding dairy and refined carbohydrates as a hardship. You will need to limit these foods in your pregnancy, so see it as practice, doing it in advance so you get pregnant and have a healthy baby.

Baby Food

Try to abstain from alcohol while planning to conceive, as even one glass of wine a week can disrupt fertility. Just two units of alcohol a week can increase levels of the sex hormone prolactin, which can adversely affect hormone balance. Fizzy drinks are full of caffeine and diet drinks contain artificial sweeteners, which are also detrimental to conception.[12]

Essential supplements to take pre-conception include 400 mg of folic acid, as it is essential for the formation and function of female sex hormones. You also need 15 mg of zinc daily, as it regulates female hormonal imbalances and is vital for the growth and correct cell division of a growing foetus. Zinc deficiency slows down the production of good eggs for conception. Foods rich in zinc include almonds, pumpkin seeds, and prawns.

Evidence shows that smoking impairs conception. Smokers have a 28 per cent lower success rate with IVF than non-smokers. Stopping smoking will improve your ability to get pregnant, decrease the chance of miscarriage, and help ensure you have a healthy baby. Smoking is bad for ovarian health. Your partner also needs to stop smoking, as it can dramatically affect the quality of sperm and lower sperm count. The British Medical Association says that 120,000 British men were rendered impotent by smoking in just one year.[13]

Some drugs, including diuretics, antibiotics, and painkillers negatively affect fertility. Painkillers can disrupt ovulation and deplete the body's store of essential nutrients. Lubricant jellies can kill off 70 per cent of sperm. Decongestant medicine can adversely affect the body's secretions, and even wearing tampons can alter the mucus in the vaginal tract.

---

12 http://infertility.health-info.org/fertility-diet-lifestyle/things-to-avoid.html
http://www.fertilityproregistry.com/article/8-foods-to-avoid-if-youre-trying-to-conceive.html
13 http://news.bbc.co.uk/1/hi/health/3477075.stm

Finally, try to sleep at night rather than stay up late and then sleep late in the morning. Our bodies work on a cycle that is designed so that we sleep when it's dark and remain awake when it's light. People who routinely stay awake through the night, such as shift workers, find that it can affect their hormones, so if you have to do shift work, try to arrange it so that leading up to conception your body is back on a 'sleeping at night and awake during the day timetable.'

Don't keep your laptop or mobile charging by the bed, and keep electrical appliances four to seven feet away from you. That includes cordless telephones and radio alarm clocks. Keep a normal phone handset by the bed and a small battery alarm clock, as the electrical magnetic frequencies emitted from all electrical appliances can have a detrimental effect on your health. When you sleep, you are stationary, so the EMFs are passing through your body for many hours.

I know I am asking you to make a lot of changes, but it will be worth it when you have your baby. The changes are not forever, and the more you can accept, and even welcome them, the easier it will be. Rather than thinking of all the foods you may have to give up, focus on all the wonderful foods you can eat that will influence your baby's taste buds and preferences, too. Remember that a mother's diet affects not only her growing baby but her baby's offspring as well. A simple way to eat to get and stay pregnant is to have eggs for breakfast (a three-egg omelette with spinach or other vegetables is ideal) or oats or plain yogurt with added nuts and seeds to increase good protein. Lunch and dinner should be based around chicken, fish, meat or lentils with vegetables and salad. Snacks should be nuts, seeds, and fruit. Eggs are the purest and most complete food in the world, after breast milk, they contain everything to create life and you can safely eat several every day.

Baby Daddy for Expectant Fathers: How to have super-elite SAS sperm.

Recent studies have shown an alarming drop in both quality and quantity of sperm, particularly in young men. They also show that sperm counts have dropped by almost a third across the Western world.[14] Sperm production is believed to be first affected in the womb, while males are developing, and then later in life by lifestyle and environmental factors. Studies today have shown modern infertility to be 40 per cent a male problem. However, there are many things men can do to improve sperm quality, quantity, and motility, including: taking supplements, altering diet, making some important lifestyle changes and visualisation techniques (I have a CD /download that helps men by using visualisation methods to increase both the quality and quantity of their sperm). It takes seventy days for sperm to form and another thirty for them to mature, so start your programme to improve sperm immediately. In order to have superior and plentiful sperm with good motility (the ability to swim well and straight), men need to take a daily dose of the following supplements:

- 10 mg of manganese daily to make sperm better swimmers.

- 30 mg of zinc, essential for healthy sperm-about forty per cent of infertile couples show that the man is deficient in zinc, and men lose zinc every time they ejaculate.

- 4,000 mcg of folic acid to improve the quality of sperm.

- 1,000 mg of vitamin B12 to improve sperm count and motility. This is especially important for men who are vegetarian or vegan.

---

14 http://www.ispub.com/journal/the-internet-journal-of-urology/volume-2-number-1/the-sperm-count-has-been-decreasing-steadily-for-many-years-in-western-industrialised-countries-is-there-an-endocrine-basis-for-this-decrease.htm

- 100 IUs of vitamin E to improve sperm activity, and also it may help the sperm penetrate the egg.
- 50 to 90 mg coenzyme Q10. ICSI fertilisation rates often rise when taking coenzyme Q10. It improves blood flow and seminal fluid, and protects sperm from free radical damage. It also gives sperm energy and increases sperm motility.

In addition, take 2,000 mg of essential fatty acids, which are crucial when trying to conceive. EFAs act as hormone regulators, and sperm should contain high concentrations of omega-3, in particular DHA (found in oily fish). DHA is in the sperm tail and helps motility and the longer the sperm tail the faster it swims. A study at the University of Copenhagen found that the sperm of men with high levels of vitamin D moved faster.

Both parents should take 100 mcg of selenium this is crucial for the development of strong, properly shaped sperm. Men need to eat bananas daily for the potassium, Brazil nuts for the selenium and drink more water to improve the seminal fluid.

Smoking damages the sperm membrane and increases the number of abnormally shaped sperm. Tobacco also reduces sperm count, its mobility and affects the sperm's ability to reach the egg. The chemical ingredient in marijuana is very closely related to testosterone, so the body will produce less of the male hormone needed for healthy sperm, if a man smokes marijuana.

In a recent Italian study, men wearing tight underwear were found to be twice as likely to be infertile as those wearing loose briefs. Male reproductive organs are external, and the scrotal skin is deliberately thin to keep sperm cooler than body temperature. The body has a normal temperature of thirty-seven degrees Celsius, but sperm functions best at thirty-two degrees Celsius, or 89.6 degrees Fahrenheit. Long distance driving, hot baths, saunas, hot tubs, tight fitting underwear or jeans, and athletic support straps, can all raise the temperature of the scrotum, thus overheating the sperm and making them ineffective.

Wearing loose underwear and taking cooler baths, avoiding saunas, and keeping the hot laptop computer off your lap, will help to keep sperm cool. Higher temperatures, even if temporary, can damage sperm. If you must work with your laptop on your legs, put a thick cushion underneath it to shield your groin from the direct heat. Don't carry your mobile in your front trouser pockets either, as mobile phones are a source of heat. Sitting behind the wheel of a car for extended periods also overheats the testes.

Excessive alcohol can have a toxic effect on sperm and will lower the sperm count, while the hops in beer and lager contain plant oestrogens, which can trigger infertility in men. Alcohol interferes with the secretion of testosterone and speeds up the conversion of testosterone into oestrogen. The breakdown product of alcohol in the body is acetaldehyde, which is toxic to sperm. Stopping, or cutting down on drinking, pre-conception, is important, as it gives the body enough time to repair itself.

Although mums-to-be are advised to eliminate coffee, for expectant fathers a little coffee (maximum two cups a day) can have a stimulating effect on sperm. The University of Sao Paulo found men who drink coffee have faster sperm.

It is important to take on all these changes with a positive attitude rather than get stressed about them. If you feel excited about the changes, you will welcome them rather than resist them. The testes become malnourished when the body is under constant stress, because the body sends blood as a priority to vital organs, like the lungs, heart, and brain and ignores the testes when stressed. The calmer you are, the more nourished your testes will be, so your sperm will be healthier, and your resulting baby will be perfectly healthy.

"The secret of success is doing ordinary things extraordinarily well."

Jim Rohn.

STEP NINE:

Baby Tunes

I once saw a client who spoke hardly any English. I work overseas with a number of Arabic women, and some of them tell me they have to get pregnant, and have sons, in order to stay married. They can't use donor eggs or sperm because their religion forbids it. This particular client was in London having IVF. Her consultant asked me if I could help her to relax before her procedure, as she was nervous, anxious, and tearful. Because conversation was difficult even with an interpreter, I downloaded Phil Spector's *Be My Baby* onto her phone and asked her to sing it every day, and her interpreter also found some equivalent songs in Arabic for her to sing to the embryo. I really was not sure how it would work, but I needed to give her something to do and to focus on while she went through the various procedures, because being anxious and nervous is detrimental to IVF. Her consultant believed that the rapid mood swings from being tense and nervous to weepy and anxious would be disastrous to her progress. I knew that if she could sing or hum her own little song throughout each procedure it would relax her and make her feel more positive. She later sent me a message via another client to say she had sung to her baby throughout the IVF procedures and the resulting pregnancy, and now had a much-loved son. Interestingly, musicians often say that when their children are born they recognise the music their parents were working on while they were in the womb. In some tribes, pregnant women carry a little bell and ring it whenever they feel particularly peaceful and happy. After their baby is born, whenever the baby is fretting, they ring the same bell and it calms the baby down because the sound carries with it the memory of hearing it in the womb when they were at their most peaceful.

I am a great believer in singing to your unborn baby. Some tribes sing to women when they are in labour, they invite and welcome the unborn baby into the world. At times I have had clients pick particular songs to sing to the baby that they wish to conceive. My absolute favourites, because of the lyrics, are:

'Baby Come to Me' by Patti Labelle.
'Be My Baby' by Phil Spector.
'Baby, I Love You' by the Ronettes.
'When a Child Is Born' by Johnny Mathis.
'Always Be My Baby' by Mariah Carey.

Singing to the baby every day is taking positive action. It is a way of connecting to the baby and having faith in its arrival. You don't need to be true to the song's lyrics. I want you to adapt them to suit you.

BABY STORIES

All the following stories and case histories are interesting and relevant. As you read through them you may find yourself identifying with a particular case, if you do simply keep reminding yourself that this is no longer you. You no longer think those thoughts or hold those beliefs so you are now free to have your baby.

Jane came to see me after suffering with unexplained infertility for several years. In her session she recalled having to look after her very ill baby brother from the age of twelve onwards. She sometimes had to leave school early to care for him and could not go to after school activities with her friends. Jane hated the responsibility and the fact that he cried so much and could not be consoled. While having to look after this fractious, unhappy baby, her thoughts were, 'I don't want any of this responsibility. It's too much for me, and it's not fair. It's not my choice to do this.' She was still thinking this same thought, subconsciously, thirty years later, and still linking thoughts of unhappiness and all the things you miss out on while raising a child, which is why she could not get pregnant. Once she had uncovered these thoughts, she got pregnant very quickly.

If you had to spend a lot of time looking after younger brothers or sisters remember you were a child then and they were not your children, they were your siblings. Looking after your own child, as a grown up woman, is different, more fulfilling and rewarding in every way, than looking after other people's children when you were still a child yourself.

Karen was only ten when she saw her baby brother die in her mother's arms, only a few weeks after he was born. Her mother was devastated by the death of her son, and Karen was never allowed to mention him, as it upset her mother so much. This left Karen unable to ever express or deal with the trauma she felt at losing her baby brother. The only memory Karen had of babies and birth was of her brother's very traumatic death and the grief it caused her mother. This left Karen fearful of having to go through what her mother went through. She was scared that she too would have a sick baby, so we used hypnosis to visualise a robust, strong baby and to make her believe that she could influence her baby's conception and development, so her baby would be strong and thriving. I saw her just before the baby was due, and she was huge. I said to her, 'That's no accident you have made such a strong, big baby,' and she had. Her baby weighed nine pounds and was like a little sumo wrestler. He was so robust, and she made that happen. Her second son was born two years later and was another big, bouncing, robustly healthy baby.

If you have been in a similar unfortunate situation it's very important to remember that you cannot repeat your mother's birth experiences, even if you want to. Medicine is hugely advanced now and you can have a healthy robust baby by influencing your mind so that your baby develops perfectly.

Rachel's first baby died at birth, she was grief stricken, had not been able to conceive again, had been feeling suicidal about her baby's death and her failure to get pregnant again. She read about my success rate in a magazine and came to see me. I explained to her that the guilt over her lost daughter and her inability to talk about it were blocking her ability to conceive. Once she had released the guilt she got pregnant immediately and had a perfect little girl followed by a perfect little boy.

If you have lost a child and are grief stricken it helps to remember that the baby you lost would want you to have another baby and to be happy. Talk about your feelings so you can let them go and imagine the child you lost sending your new baby to you and being delighted that you are able to experience a happy wonderful pregnancy and birth.

Susan had been pregnant in her teens and had undergone an abortion, which she kept secret from her family. She felt such guilt about terminating her pregnancy and believed that she did not deserve to have another baby. She was in effect punishing herself by not allowing herself to get pregnant again. We used hypnosis to let go of this, and Susan became pregnant and had a baby within a year of her appointment with me.

All humans make mistakes you are allowed to get something wrong but not to punish your own body by denying yourself children. The baby you did not have, because of circumstances that were not your fault, would want you to have another baby and to be happy. When you make a mistake and learn from it you have improved your character and you are automatically forgiven, because you are not the same person you were then. Imagine the child you lost sending your new baby to you and being delighted that you are able to experience a happy wonderful pregnancy and birth.

Julia had a very cold, distant mother and felt quite excluded from the relationship her parents had together. She felt ignored and left out throughout her childhood. Her father had idolised her mother, and Julia always felt that she was in the way. When Julia married, she felt it was the first time someone loved her just as she was. Her husband adored her, but on some level this reminded her of her parent's relationship, and Julia feared that when she had a baby she might resent it just as her mother had resented her. Or her husband might love the baby more than he loved her, and as a result her only experience of being the most important person in the world to one person would be over forever. Once she identified this, she was able to see the differences between her and her mother, as well as her husband and her father. The fear was released, and she had a baby very easily, followed by a second child a year later.

Remind yourself of how very different you are to your parents and how much love you will give to your baby. You have given so much time and effort into conceiving this chid and it will always feel loved, cherished and valued by you. Often when our own parents are not loving enough we are so aware of how wrong that feels and this, in turn, can make us better and more loving parents more attuned to our child's needs.

Victoria was a very interesting case as she did not menstruate at all and, despite undergoing medical and fertility treatment, she still did not have periods. When we talked about this I asked her to tell me what her early periods were like and she replied that 'she got them at 13 and thought they were disgusting and she hated having them'. She was the first girl in her class to get them and felt embarrassed and different to her friends. She had painful cramps and a heavy bleed and recalled taking to her bed on several occasions when her relatives were visiting and feeling so resentful that she could not be downstairs enjoying the occasion. She remembered wishing that she did not have periods and loathing everything about them. She stopped menstruating within two years and by the time Victoria went to college her periods were non-existent. She described sharing a house with several other girls at college who all complained about their monthly bleeds while she simply never had them. She was very involved in sport at college and considered it such an asset to be period free that when she walked past sanitary products she would feel smug and delighted that they were something that did not concern her. Once she could see how her mind linked pain and disgust to menstruating she was able to begin a different dialogue with her mind. Recognising that the feelings she had, at only thirteen, were very different to the feelings she had now. She chose to feel excited about the bleeds and pleased that her body functioned in the way a healthy woman's body is meant to function. She even chose to feel delighted about buying tampons and within four weeks she had a light bleed, followed the next month by a full period, and four months later she was pregnant and is now a mother of two.

I have worked with many women whose first pregnancy failed because the amniotic fluid was lost or because the lungs did not develop or the heart stopped and many other sad scenarios. With each of these women I had them imagine the amniotic fluid staying for nine months and the lungs developing perfectly and the heart working perfectly throughout their pregnancy. In each instance their second pregnancy was perfect with no repeat of what happened in the earlier one. If you have been unfortunate enough to experience any abnormalities with a previous pregnancy you can imagine the opposite happening in your next pregnancy. Using your knowledge and imagination tell your baby to develop perfectly and see the opposite of what happened in the earlier pregnancy so that this one is textbook perfect.

"What lies behind us and what lies before us are tiny matters compared to what lies within us."

Ralph Waldo Emerson.

STEP TEN:

Baby Shower

Well done! You have finished the book and made many changes that can only help you. Let's just recap on all the great things you have done, and are going to continue to do on your way to becoming a mother.

Baby Book

You should have a notebook, what I like to call a baby book, where you can look at all the things you wrote as you worked through this programme. You have written in it all your reasons for having a baby and why you will be a wonderful mother. Write down why you know that no baby in the world will be more loved and wanted than your baby. No baby will come into the world with more of a sense of knowing it was meant to be here, and that it has a right to be here. Your baby will have a meaning and a purpose, and that is a wonderful gift for any child to go through life with. One of the best things you can give your baby is for it to know it was planned and wanted. Imagine when your baby is older, talking about its journey to be born, and showing them your book. Children love to hear over and over about what it was like when they were growing in your tummy and what it was like when they were born and how happy everyone was. So imagine telling them that story as they sit on your knee, and showing them your book and all the things you did to make sure your baby was born to *you*. When my daughter was about five, she asked me to draw a picture of the best day of my life. I drew a little picture of me sitting up in a hospital bed holding my baby, and I drew a little chart clipped to the end of the bed that said 'baby Phaedra Peer.' She was delighted by the picture, because it validated how significant and important she was to me, and she has kept it to this day.

Baby Steps

You know the power of visualisation and how important it is to see yourself as a mother and to accept yourself as a parent. When parents are very close to adoption, they begin buying baby things as opposed to avoiding the baby aisles and baby shops. They get their future child's room ready and talk about their child. The brain receives a very clear message: she's having a baby, she's becoming a parent, she is a mother and consequently that is exactly what she becomes. The strongest force is the mind, and the body has to mirror, honour, and match what is going on in it. It cannot be a coincidence that so many women conceive naturally after adoption, or after an IVF baby. It occurs because finally they accept, and see themselves, as a mother.

Baby Shopping

Go down the baby aisles in the supermarket and into the baby shops, and plan all the things you will buy. Touch, smell, and feel the items. Look through baby catalogues, and plan your baby's room, wardrobe, and nursery. Buy some socks or a little hat as faith that your baby is on its way to you. Women who are not conceiving tend to avoid baby shops and baby areas, whereas couples waiting for IVF and adoption often fall pregnant during the process because they see and accept themselves as parents, expecting a baby. The rate of natural conception after IVF and adoption is quite high,[15] as the couples now feel like a family. Their brains accept that they are parents and the issue of infertility is closed. Infertile couples are asked to use birth control for up to three years after adoption due to the high statistics of adoptive parents conceiving. Accept yourself as a mother-to-be. You *are* an expectant mother as you do this programme.

Baby Talk

Talk to your baby every single day. Welcome your baby into your womb, into your home, into your life, and into your heart. Send love to your baby; let it know how much you want it. Describe to the baby all the things you will do together and as a family. Show your baby that it's wanted. Show it all the flowers, cards, gifts, and balloons that greet you as you bring your baby home from hospital, as well as the aunties, uncles, grandparents, cousins, and friends who are so excited about welcoming your baby into the world. Talk to your baby and show it how you imagine it will be as you enjoy all the firsts...the first tooth, the first crawl, the first steps, the first paddle in the sea, the first Christmas, the first birthday, the first holiday and the first day at school. Invite your baby into your life to share these wonderful moments and experiences with you.

---

15   http://www.heraldsun.com.au/news/more-news/after-ivf-babies-just-come-naturally/story-e6frf7kx-1111115300192

Baby Love

When you have sex, imagine conception taking place. Try watching the movie *Look who's Talking,* for a fun idea of what takes place at conception. Talk to your baby, and tell it to begin its journey to be born to you now. Imagine a perfect egg drawing a perfect sperm towards it, perfect fertilisation taking place, and your fertilised egg becoming a foetus, implanting securely in your womb, and growing on target for nine months.

Baby Face

See your baby. You don't need a crystal clear image. You can see your baby in profile, or as a new-born or a foetus, or as a toddler. Talk to it every day.

Baby Shower

Shower your baby with love and positive thoughts. Send it white healing light to keep it strong and safe and healthy in your womb. Maintain a really healthy diet and the right vitamins to boost conception, and imagine you are already a wonderful mother doing everything for your baby.

Baby Power

Your egg is intelligent. It contains a life force all of its own, and it knows exactly what to do at every stage of conception. If you show it, instruct it, command it, and rehearse with it what is to happen, your egg will do it. Women with only one ovary have eggs that are so smart, they swim to and then travel down the alternate fallopian tube every other month.

Baby House
See your baby's presence everywhere...the cot in the baby room, the baby basket in your room, the baby bath and all the baby products in the bathroom, the highchair and sterilising unit in the kitchen, the playpen in the lounge, the buggy in the hall, the car seat in the car, the paddling pool, sandpit and swing in the garden, toys and teddies everywhere. Take the baby on a tour of your house. Show it how wanted and loved it is, where it will sleep, play, eat, bathe, and how much love is waiting for it in your home.

Baby Sensations
Throughout IVF, visualise each procedure and every medication taking you closer to your baby. Welcome and celebrate each step. End every visualisation with the same image of you holding your baby in your arms in your hospital bed. Before and during any medical procedure, such as egg collection or embryo transfer, remind yourself that in nine months you will be in another bed in a similar room delivering your baby. Talk to your baby, and tell it this.

Baby Care
You are a wonderful, loving mother. You are great parents, and you bond with your baby immediately. You instinctively know what to do...rocking, patting, singing to your baby, speaking in a low soothing voice. You are a natural mother, and you love raising your child. See images of you and your baby bathing together or snuggled up in bed together.

Misconceptions

They are everywhere in the field of fertility. There is a lot of information in this book designed to help you to become a mother, but please don't feel you have to be perfect and rigid in your approach to making your baby. Relax, and do as much as you can without becoming fanatical.

It's important to balance the things this book asks you to do while eliminating stress as much as possible. Don't fret if you can't always find organic food, or if you have an off day. Just do what you can, as much as you can, while believing this is helping you to make your baby.

It is essential that you have not only read this book from cover to cover but that you have done all of the exercises required (if you have skipped any please go back and do them right now, not for me but for you). I wrote this book to help you have a baby so please do the exercises. From the beginning to the end of this book you have been absorbing powerful workable techniques to improve your fertility. If you adhere to this programme and use this book the way it was meant to be used you will get results.

Baby Shower

I hope you have enjoyed this journey towards motherhood. Thank you so much for taking it with me and I wish you every success. Please keep in touch with me and let me know of your progress. You can email me for advice at info@marisapeer.com or contact me at www.tryingtogetpregnant.co.uk I would love you to send me a picture of your baby so I can add it to all the photos on my baby wall of children who came into the world because of the techniques in this book.

Love from,

Marisa Peer

Marisa Peer was named Best British Therapist *by Men's Health magazine* and features *in Tatler's Guide* to Britain's 250 Best Doctors. She has spent 25 years working with an extensive client list including royalty, rock stars, actors, professional and Olympic athletes, CEOs and media personalities and has developed her own style that is frequently referred to as life-changing. Marisa is a best-selling author of four books and appears extensively, as an expert, on television and radio including Channel 4's Supersize vs. Superskinny and ITV's Celebrity Fit Club UK and Celebrity Fit Club USA. She is the nutritionist for Men's Fitness magazine and the therapist in the Sunday People's Heart to Heart column and has her own weekly Mind column for Closer Magazine.

Printed in Great Britain
by Amazon